FIBROSUCCESS

Fibromyalgia Explained, Managed and Eliminated

Dearest Esme + Harry,
Best to you - you have watched me grow up all these years, now I am a writer to share with the world + those closest to me!
Jemma Jackson

FIBROSUCCESS

Fibromyalgia Explained, Managed and Eliminated

*One woman's journey to find a
Solution
to help Doctors and Patients*

by

Jemma Jacksen
RCT   CCT   BSc

FIBROSUCCESS
Copyright @ 2013 by Jemma Jacksen
All Rights Reserved

Self Published

This book is intended as a reference book only, not as a medical manual. I make no claims to an actual cure.

The information herein is designed to help you make better informed decisions about your health and wellness. It is not intended as a substitute for any treatment that my have been or will be prescribed by your doctor(s). If you suspect you have a medical condition, I urge you to seek competent and capable medical help.

Mention of specific companies, authorities or organizations in this book does not imply endorsement by the author, nor does mention of specific companies, authorities or organizations imply they endorse this book or it's author.

Internet addresses and sources mentioned in this book were accurate at the time it was published.
Any characters or scenarios which may seem similar are mere coincidences.

No part of this book may be used or reproduced or copied in any manner or form whatsoever with out prior written permission of the author. Copyright 2015.

ISBN : 978-0-9921405-0-2
Printed and bound in Canada 2013, 2015

All Artwork By Jemma : www.jemmajacksen.com
1st Edition October 10, 2013
2nd Edition January 16, 2015
3 rd Edition May 10, 2015

Dedication:

" to all those who suffer mentally and/or physically especially alone or in the dark"

and

"to all the people who have helped me in life- you know who you are,..... in particular my mom and Rob for playing a big part in this books existence"

and

Bosley

"The more I endure, the better I get at enduring it "
(Jemma)

CONTENTS:

FIBROSUCCESS

Fibromyalgia Explained, Managed and Eliminated

TABLE OF CONTENTS   Page 7

i. Disclaimer.   Page 12
ii. Preface (forward)   Page 15
    INTRO   Page 17

PART 1 : FIBRO EXPLAINED   **20**

I. All about Fibromyalgia and Doctors view.   20
   pain, fatigue and inflammation, immune system.
   -Leaky Gut Syndrome   24
  – The Amygdala: it's role in fibro- trauma, nerves,   26
        fight/flight

II. About me and my Symptoms of Fibro.,   31
   how long.

III. My Experimenting with Fixes and Mg.   34

IV. Facts about Magnesium and Ca.   38

V. **Why Women more affected than Men.**   **43**
    Estrogen and hormonal imbalances   44
    Estrogen and the Brain   45
    Hormones   48
    -**Adrenal burnout** & Hormones   49

VI. **WHY MG WORKS IN MY OPINION.**   **56**

    -Calcium and Aging   60
    -Magnesium Sources   60
    - other diseases Mg can help with   62

    WARNING : TOO MUCH Mg   63

VII. **GLUTEN**: (inflammation- gluten riddance)   **65**
    "the gluten connection"   65
    Inflammation   71
    My Story with Gluten   74
    Wheat and the Brain   75
    Gluten and the Tummy   76

PART 2 : FIBRO MANAGED   81

VIII.   **Fibro Symptoms and Vitamins that Work.**   81- 115

page
81   Depression
84   Should you be on Anti-depressants ?
87   Medications Vs. Natural Remedies for Depression
91   Stress "Stress is Contagious"
92   - Nurturing our own Bodies
95   Mental Stress
98   Emotional Health connected to Physical Health

101	Stigma with depression - "Stigma sucks"
104	Mood
106-112	Fatigue (culprits- Anemia, Insomnia, Wt. Gain, Depression, Thyroid problems, Candida yeast overgrowth, Mitral valve prolapse, Gluten)
112	Energy Boosters
114	Pain
115	Ischemia & Pain

VIIII. FEELINGS/ ENERGY IS CONTAGIOUS   117

"thoughts are feelings, feelings are Energy"

PART 3 : FIBRO ELIMINATED   126

X **My Prescription (diet) to help alleviate, Eliminate fibro**. 126

Magnesium discussed	127
(chemical rxns involved in, symptoms of deficiency, test for deficiency, what Mg helps with)	
Diet (What I do)	134
Cost	135
easy steps	136
Story Board- tell your story	138
As well what I do	139
What I recommend	141
Resolve	142
Warning too much Mg	146
Concluding Thoughts	150
Summary diagram	154 & 155
How Fibro crept back into my life	156

XI. Who is right, the MD or Naturopath? 158
(Western medicine vs. Eastern medicine)

XII CONCLUSION 160

PART 4

XIII DEPRESSION - in more detail 163-173
Why it happens, how to help it
Probiotics and the brain 163

PART 5

XIIII RANDOM RELATED TOPICS 174-280

page
174 Why I wrote this Book
176 Change
178 Sexual Abuse/Physical Abuse
180 How we feel about Others in our Life (having a mate)
182 Vulnerability, Rejection and Bullying
187 Sadness and Grief
189 Those on Disability
190 Self Worth
194 Destiny
195 Relationships are like playing lotto 649
197 Water
198 Pacing Ourselves
200 Life is a Canvas
202 Suffering
204 Working and how we treat the disabled
206 The Heart (Heart failure and disease)
209 Weight Loss

212	Hormones
216	Addictions
218	Get over it! (injury and trauma)
221	Hormones and Diet
223	The Brain
225	People's Perceptions of Others (Fear, Ego, Jealousy)
232	Jealousy, vengeance and being called Crazy
236	Climb That Mountain !
241	"Lets Talk about it"
244	Food Sensitivities- Why we are such an angry nation
245	We all do it- We judge
247	Self – Love
248	When our Hearts Break Over a Loss
252	God will light the way (random thoughts)
254	Fear, Anger and Self- Pity
256	Accept Different
259	Live in the Light not the Dark
262	Truth
269	Don't take Offence
273	Create Love
275	Similar circumstances, two completely different Outcomes
277	We all need Goliaths
281	A Word about Families

XV. References and Sources   283

ABOUT THE AUTHOR   285

Contact INFO   287

Disclaimer:

This book is not to be used as a substitute for appropriate medical care and consultation, nor should any information in it be interpreted as prescriptive. Any persons who suspect they have a medical problem or disease should consult their physicians for guidance and proper treatment.

This is purely only my "opinion" based on both my extensive experience with Fibromyalgia and my education in science (pre-med and RCT) and my bit of reading. So pretty much fiction (borderline nonfiction), I make no claims here of cures or resolution of Fibromyalgia, only an educated guess. I hope it helps even just one person even tho I'm only a trial of 1. Become your own doctor, you can. Good luck and happy reading.

For serious medical problems and/or questions please consult a local physician or specialist.

"the two most important days in ones life is the day you are born and the day you figure out Why"
(Mark Twain)

" Pain is inevitable, suffering is Optional"
..... (author unknown, some say buddha)

TO
Accomplish
Great Things
WE
Must Not
ONLY
ACT
but Also
DREAM
not Only
PLAN
but Also
BELIEVE

FIBROSUCCESS:
Fibromyalgia Explained, Managed and Eliminated

Fibro: "fibers"
myalgia: "muscle pain"

PREFACE:

In this book I outline what Fibromyalgia is, how it possibly exists and why and how one can manage and eventually eliminate it, like I did. It covers alot about my experience with Fibromyalgia. The methods are simple to do, follow and inexpensive and I am not selling or promoting any products. I mention ones I believe in thru experience, I am not biased. I talk about how the remedies may work or help.

The book is quite simple and a short, easy read. The concepts are easily understood I hope. I discuss doctors point of view and how to deal with them and which one to pick for yourself to help you. I believe a good doctor will work WITH you as a ``TEAM``. I discuss STRESS ALOT and how it impacts this illness, fatigue and depression as well as a bit about Gluten, and most importantly DIET and how these all play a role.

I also discuss why I think women are more impacted than men by this illness. This book is general in a way and very much in layman terms, I do not claim to be an acclaimed writer (or physician) so it is not meant to win any writing awards but is rather alot of tried and true and ``make sense information`` from someone who has a BALANCED opinion and much experience in dealing with Fibromyalgia.

Fibromyalgia is like no other illness, you cannot see it, it is often not believed or understood and alot of doctors see it as new and a trend as well as thinking ``it is all in your head``, I know you have heard your share of that! The illness deals with the body AND the head and I discuss fully here how to help both at the same time. It pours out all my secrets, thoughts and realizations on this topic and I hope people find it of value and that I did not waste my time, even tho this writing gave me good practice!

So go ahead and read on and I hope it flows for you and the info sticks, always be your own doctor because you know you best and be proactive in your health, for without health, a person has absolutely NOTHING! *This book is not intended to replace practical medical advice.* My hope is this book gives you ALOT to help you and I help contribute. From one that is now better, I hope it helps you.

2/3 rds of this book explores Fibromyalgia (and stress) and the other 1/3 rd discusses mind, body, spirit issues surrounding depression and long term illness.

INTRO: FIBROSUCCESS

Fibromyalgia is for the most part much a mystery as so few have really taken time out of their lives to figure it out and if so, write about it and share it. All opinions help solve problems I believe. Mine is but one opinion but I believe a good one and makes sense.

This book is easy to read, flows well I hope from topic to topic and for one with Fibro will be easily understood. I have picked up a couple Fibro books to scan over (preview) and they are filled with complicated theories, formulas, assumptions and complexity. I understand how hard it is for one with Fibro to read, understand and even retain info so I am unsure why these books were even written that way and I found for myself, with a science background and degree hard to follow them or swallow. Not many points I could take away from them and so thick too! Hundreds of pages. Then I believe there is a smaller one out there but I never saw and didn't wish to find as I want my ideas my own and not lean towards others thoughts on the topic. This thin book I just mentioned is probably too thin and scantily covers the topic, I dunno.

My book on the other hand is short enough and long enough and most importantly very simple. Simple to look up topics and simple to relate to. I cover many topics off the wall that people deal with having Fibro. (non-scientific). I give my full regime, simple to follow at the end. I believe it is very relatable and user friendly.

Some people feel fibromyalgia is a label or rather "umbrella" that some specific diseases just fall under. That Fibro and it's symptoms are too general and covers many specific illnesses. This may well be or seem true, however I feel it's that these illnesses, that all fall under the "umbrella" are all somehow linked and affect each other. That is my approach. Some feel people are labelled Fibro when in fact they may simply have vitamin deficiency, it be toxicity environmentally or something viral or trauma induced. I feel all these are linked together and in helping one you help them all eventually. What one needs to focus on is removing the cause that is making the body so weak to issues like toxicity. If a person is strong and healthy they will have less sensitivities and/or allergies and be able to fight viruses. I feel the main focus is DIET- nutrition- for what we put into our bodies is so very Important. Most important thing and place to start is DIET but what is equally important is IF our food is even being absorbed or utilized properly. It is one thing to get enough of something but if your body doesn't use it and it goes right thru you – it does not help any. So in affect you need to repair the body and get it in healthy working order to absorb and utilize the DIET you feed it. This means a healthy gut! **Immunity, and serotonin production and all disease starts with the gut. 90% of the immune system is in the gut.**

I take a holistic approach in my book in looking at simultaneously healing the mind, body and spirit, as you heal one, you heal the other as they are all connected and cannot exist alone. They need balance and healthy balance. SO in this book you will find methods to help your physical body and methods to help your mind and also topics covering spirit. They all go together and is not hard to implement daily, working on all at the same time. As one area gets stronger it will help strengthen the others. This approach is unique to this book.

Some believe if you have fibro to go see your naturopath. I feel this is a good idea in order to get some specifics and especially if the methods in my book don't help you at all. A good naturopath will help pinpoint your cause and possibly inform you that you have another problem instead of fibro. I have not heard alot of stories about Naturopaths resolving or curing fibro, just in "management" of the ailment. But certainly they are useful and you may find quite helpful, if you can afford it. They may run tests on you and get some answers. I fear they will mainly work on the physical though, you would need to see a guru or therapist to work on the spiritual/mind part. That is why I feel my book would work so well for those suffering, I focus on physical and mental simultaneously and by the end tell you why this is so important and how to start solving it and unravelling the illness one step at a time.

FIBROSUCCESS

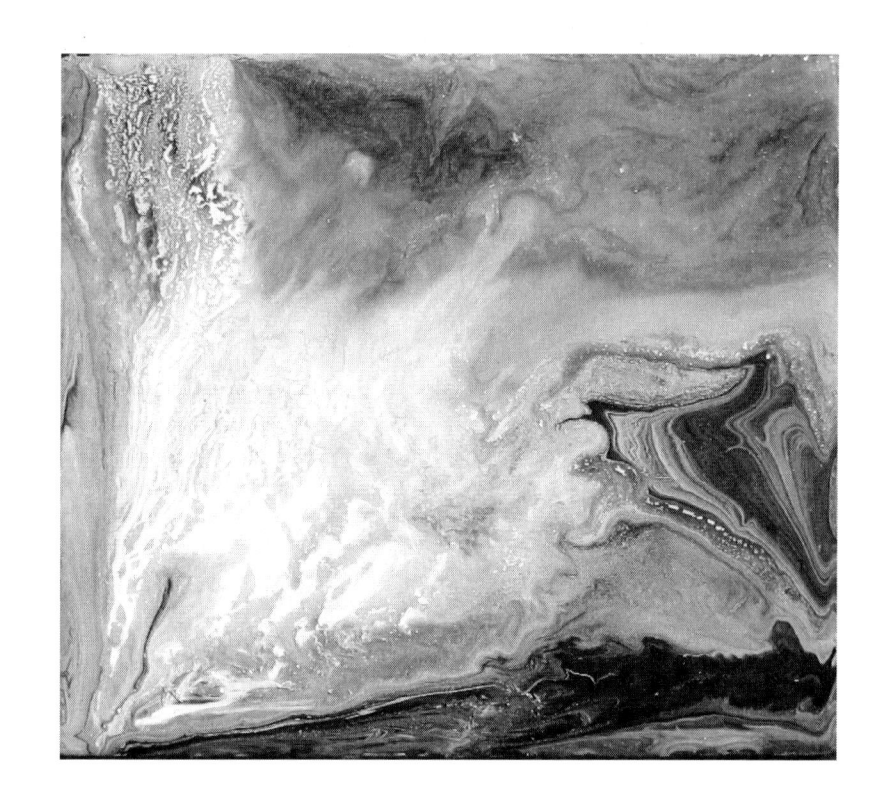

PART 1- FIBRO EXPLAINED

I. All About Fibro and the Doctors View.

Pain / Fatigue and Inflammation / Immune System.
"Leaky Gut Syndrome"
The Amygdala

I know all about Fibromyalgia- the fatigue, aches and pains all over for no reason, the foggy brain, the depression and anxiety and all the allergies and sensitivities. Sometimes I'd just lay in bed so tired and hurting I could not fall asleep. The memory or rather "lack of"- can't remember or put together the simplest thoughts. Feels like dementia. I thought I had dementia. I told my doctor I thought I had dementia and he laughed at me "no you don't " he replied. Not the first time he has laughed. Well it feels like it I said. Don't get me wrong, nothing against doctors here but they are like any other profession, the good ones and the bad ones. I like the ones that care and will look into it.

My Fibro really kicked in last June 2010 so I've had it real bad for just two years now. Mainly due to stress I figured. I just finished 3 years of schooling and had a major exam to complete my diploma in Cardiology Technology. The weather doesn't help either- damp and cool as I live in Vancouver, BC Canada and have for the past 25 years now. The pressure changes play havoc with Fibro. On an overcast day expect alot of fatigue and pain unrelieved by anything. I could predict the weather better than any meteorologist by now. When it is clear and sunny and warm, no real complaints.

I am now 45 years old and may have had CFS/ Fibro in my early 20's as I suffered mono in university and did not take good care of it (thought earlier by many to be a great link). Doctors resorted to the diagnosis of CFS, "just live with it " they'd say (specialist) and did not run any tests on me.

One specialist, while in my 20's, told me that ``we are not going to waste any money on people LIKE YOU (me) when there are heart patients in line for tests.`` So I then investigated it and this was the mid 1990's. I learned alot about it- CFS and Fibromyalgia. Maybe I had it, maybe not, as it turns out later on when I was real adamant about something more serious going on (I was extremely tired, dizzy, SOB, etc)- the Doctors did one test only because I begged and cried alot- an echo was performed on my heart. An awesome doctor said "if you are tired, it could be your heart, let's take a picture of it". (I think he just wanted me to stop crying too). The echo was not performed quickly, I got in line with everyone else.

Well, upon that test it was soon discovered the root of most my ills were due to a hole in my heart (ASD-atrial septal defect) and I needed (required) life saving open heart surgery to repair it or else I would die in a year they informed me. My heart chambers pressures were on the verge of changing for the worse. So, again in line I got for that and thought nothing ever again about CFS or Fibro until recently.

Upon my heart surgery most of my symptoms of fatigue, dizzy, memory loss, SOB etc had disappeared. Now was fibro creeping up again (?) due to stress and possibly poor diet. Maybe. Anyway going to doctors is rather interesting- most, if not all will tell you Fibro does not exist, "it is all in your head", "here are some anti-depressants and painkillers, go home" or "maybe see a therapist". No answers or even guesses. They know so little about it and believe so little. I did the regular touch test to see if I had tender spots (trigger points) but mostly the doctor just rubbed my shoulders and said yep you have Fibro- not much we can do for you. Oh brother I thought- they do not feel what I feel, I must again become my own doctor. So I did. I looked into what worked, how Fibro comes about, what triggers it and what helps relieve it (even minimally). I bought a couple immunity books but mostly went trial by error to see what worked. I had heard a few vitamins worked so I bought and tried those. Nothing. There were special concoctions for it, but again nothing. There were all these really expensive programs promising results but who has that kind of money esp. when not working, for possible witchcraft and unfounded theories. Sure they helped, maybe a little (?). I'm unsure.

Fibromyalgia is probably the most prevalent and most understudied disease/illness of our time. Strikes women more than men and I will explain in detail later why so. I will also give my opinion of how it comes about, what triggers it badly and how to possibly manage or cure it for yourself, making your life liveable again and productive. Most people don't believe in it, including doctors because there is no definitive test for it and you cannot see it like a bruise or broken arm, but it feels 10x worse, the nerves in the body and all your muscles are on high alert, and it hurts! And the fatigue feels like you've worked all week with no rest or sleep. I believe insomnia may be part of it as well so on top of being exhausted you have too much anxiety to rest the mind and fall asleep. With frustration and lack of getting anything accomplished in life one gets depressed and lonely. This is a frustrating possible side effect of Fibro. Everything is so bad health and life wise you do wish to just die and you believe you are going to.

Read on and I will explain my point of view on Fibro, my experience and how I feel much better today than I did two years ago. Fibro virtually eliminated outta my life! You don' t have to live with it or think it's all in your head because it isn't. It is real and I offer real solutions.

"Is it simply depression?"...doctors always suggested it is merely depression and the pervasive aches and pains that come with it. Well I believe it is partly depression showing up in the "ill" mind alongside the body and usually 'after' the body.

This book is intended to help those who have no answers or direction, simple things to try and if you don't have Fibro yourself, I am sure you know someone who has it and will benefit from reading this simple, yet clear and concise short book. It is easy to read.

IMPORTANT NEW TOPIC:

"LEAKY GUT SYNDROME"

(this can parade as Fibro or is it the cause?- A good question)

I will discuss briefly about leaky gut syndrome but not in detail as it is not the scope of this book but one who reads this may just have this disorder and confuse it with Fibro.

Leaky Gut Syndrome gives the same symptoms of fatigue, joint pain, depression, rash, thyroid problems and bloating. Seems more related to problems with gluten then strictly inflammation (Fibro)-maybe intertwined?.

"All disease starts in the Gut", Hypocrites once said.

One should take Omega 3's to help resolve leaky gut as well as avoid dairy, gluten and lower the sugar intake, also no potatoes, no tomatoes.

Leaky gut syndrome is essentially holes in the lining of the gut where stuff that is suppose to pass out in feces, instead goes into the blood stream and makes it's way to tissues and joints. The "holes" in the gut allow toxins and bacteria to escape and go thru into the joints causing inflammation- leads to "autoimmune disease". So very similar to Fibro in effect. Once a child was diagnosed with "adolescent idiopathic arthritis" when in fact it was discovered he really had leaky gut. Some of his symptoms were bloating, gas, cramps, skin eczema, joint pain and fatigue. The joints seem to be the biggest problem in this as things that shouldn't go thru to the blood and body do and go to the joints and cause problems. Where there exists a problem in this is that the body will attack these foreign invaders and as they lodge themselves in the tissue and joints thus the tissues and joints get attacked also, leading to this inflammation problem and pain (autoimmune disease). Nutrients are naturally suppose to get thru as they are broken down & absorbed and smaller and do not cause an issue. It is when toxins, say gluten is allowed thru for example, that is not suppose to get thru. These don't get thru if the lining protects you like it should in a healthy individual with no leaky gut.

People with this leaky gut often have food sensitivities/ allergies, antibiotic overuse, high NSAID'S (non steroidal anti-inflammatory drugs) use, high sugar diet or parasites.
The test for leaky gut is called the "intestinal permeability test" whereby the person drinks say a beaker full of water filled with sugar molecules, small molecules and bigger molecules. The urine is then tested 6 hours later, the lab determines how many small and big molecules made it in the urine, if big made it in , then leaky gut is diagnosed.

Doctors recommend 3 steps if you have leaky gut, they are :

1. "*Remove*"- **AVOID GLUTEN**, dairy, refined sugar, alcohol, egg plant, tomatoes and potatoes (avoid NSAIDS as well).
2. "*Replace*"- add good bacteria to your diet with a good **pro- biotic**.
3. "*Repair*"- help repair the lining of the gut with **omega 3's**, flax, salmon (wild), nuts, walnuts, and "Glutamine"(helps repair).

Word of warning with Glutamine tho, a friend of mine had leaky gut bad and took alot of Glutamine, it went right thru, straight to his brain and caused extreme rage and kinda psychotic behaviour. So be very careful how it affects you and start with small doses you can handle, stepping it up over time as it repairs and is thus less toxic to the brain that way. Removing gluten will make large strides in helping to repair the gut. If you do nothing else, try to eliminate almost completely this common allergen from your diet. Gluten ruins the gut and makes it nearly impossible to absorb proper nutrients from good food sources.

THE AMYGDALA

The brain is a forever changing Organ. It develops 'new neurons' coined now most aptly, "neuro- plasticity". It is important to realize here that if you do have a defect in your brain that you can heal. As it is after all an organ, able to heal itself as most other organs can. If you have chronic fatigue syndrome, Fibro, Multiple chemical sensitivity, PTSD or golf war syndrome, there is hope. Even mental illness to some degree can be resolved I believe.

Much is done through retraining the brain and a lot of meditation to make new connections but I believe deeply that nutrition and vitamins can assist, namely one mineral in particular, Magnesium. Magnesium helps calm the Amygdala which is often (I believe) in overdrive in people with Fibro and maybe other traumas.

The Amygdala…

In Brief: The Amygdala is like a battery for the car, when it is lit up, it sends signals throughout the body triggering the fight/flight reactions, it will activate all the nerves of the body. It is like the main signal centre. If "broken" due to over activation/trauma, it will send these signals and make the nerves overactive or oversensitive than regular. This is why I believe we can be sensitive to even the slightest touch, it hurts. Our sensitivity to pain is out of whack, not normal.

In detail: The Amygdala is a tiny, almond shaped neuronal structure in the brain based at the bottom of the limbic region, just above the brain stem (Kind of in the lower middle of the brain). There exists two of these little almond shaped structures(organs) in the brain, one in each hemisphere, the right and the left. The amygdala forms an integral part of the autonomic nervous system, reacting to both adrenaline and cortisol. The autonomic nervous system (ANS) is the area of the brain stem and connection that automatically regulates muscle, cardiac and glandular responses. Signals from Hormones are sent here. The amygdala is also deeply connected to the hypothalamus, a neuronal structure at the base of the limbic system that releases adrenaline and other hormones into the bloodstream, to send signals throughout the body. The emotional memories and reaction(s) the amygdala and hypothalamus create are extremely powerful, linked to significant biological and biochemical reactions throughout our bodies. Quite simply the amygdala is a powerful little thing.

The amygdala in simple terms is essentially our "fight or flight response" which we've all heard about. The amygdala interprets outside stimuli, and maybe viruses as well, to determine if they are a danger. If so, the amygdala communicates with the hypothalamus which turns on this fight or flight response, also known as the sympathetic nervous system response or simply the stress response. Thus, a bunch of biochemicals are then released into the body in reaction and some of the body systems, such as the digestive system, may shut down in order to maximize energy to respond to this supposed or real threat. Our perceptions of danger and stress duly play a major role in this response. As if we are too sensitive then it can go into overdrive quite easily. Most of the time when there is real danger then there is a normal response. Ones system is not meant to be on high alert 24/7, all the time. This is too hard on the body and most likely causes all the pain and fatigue one feels with Fibro. If put into overdrive such as people with Fibro, this protective system meant to keep us safe from bodily injury rather becomes harmful to the body. This all may adversely affect the Immune and Hormonal systems leading to all sorts of things such as headaches, Pain(all over), disruption of sleep cycles (insomnia), viral infections (as weakens immunity) and related illnesses such as IBS, CFS, Fibro, Immune disorders, Autoimmunity problems/Diseases and others.

Is it that Fibro patients are genetically predisposed by physical structure and oversensitivity that the amygdala is sent into overdrive ? Or is it that something occurs, and triggers this important part of the brain to "snap", kind of break and remain in overdrive. I'm not sure anyone has the answers yet. It may very well be a combination. I do begin to realize however that people with Fibro are usually the 'over sensitive' types. What is also common among Fibro patients as well is that a lot of them may have experienced trauma. This is part of the reason trauma such as a car accident, abuse or something viral maybe said to "overbreak" the amygdala. If one gets too much cortisol or adrenalin surging thru their body it can deeply impact this amygdala. **Too much adrenaline or cortisol is sure to damage the body. (too much meaning beyond what the body requires**).

Chronic sympathetic arousal will cause these stress chemicals to accumulate in the body. These stress chemicals are mostly adrenaline, nor adrenaline and cortisol.

I've already explained in this book, why more women are impacted than men in that men have less cortisol naturally. This makes a lot of sense then. Things such as coffee or a bad diet can increase these adrenaline and cortisol levels in both men or women though. Probably the reason why exercise negatively impacts those with Fibro– it releases amounts of adrenaline. This then could be a bit of 'adrenaline overload' for some and they feel the negative impact of pain and fatigue. I believe the amygdala can be calmed, healed and brought back to normal and what I believe is that magnesium can help this to a substantial degree. It is already known and proven that magnesium can help headaches.

Magnesium is calming to neuron's, the brain, body and muscles. Perhaps it helps block all these signals or stress hormones in the body that circulate and create pain, the heightened sensitivity of the amygdala (I believe the nerves are on high alert and this causes the pain to touch) and fatigue of the muscles. If your muscles are constantly contracting under duress like with a lot of calcium then they get worn out and tired. Magnesium counters the action of calcium. We are missing magnesium from our soils, food and water so much so that I believe sometimes Fibro can be "something in the water", or rather something missing in the water.

We need to supplement magnesium for the brain to calm itself and not be in high alert, at first possibly large supplementation then tapering to a maintenance level. This amygdala being over sensitized and broken makes Fibro a real physical condition not a psychological one. Mind you I feel we can do a lot like meditation to help, and decreasing our reactions and sensitivities to events that occur daily in our lives. A restful time for the brain allows it to rest, heal and may form new, more healthy connections. So take magnesium, especially before bed, meditate and watch your stress level, caffeine intake and thinking patterns (perceptions). **This all affects the brain physically, as emotional as it may seem, the two are intimately tied together and cannot be separated**. People especially in our Western medicine like to separate the two and treat them each as one. It is mostly in the eastern medicine that they are treated together. I believe they should be treated as one and not separated. That is why I talk about the book here as a mind, body, Spirit approach, BOTH physical and emotional situation.

I believe once the Amygdala "heals" from its broken state, like any other organ, it will thusly perform appropriately and healthy and pain and the such go away; just like the adrenals can heal.

In Brief, the amygdala is the fight & flight centre in the middle of the brain and when trauma occurs, whether it be physical or emotional, the amygdala can be triggered into overdrive. This overdrive activates all the neurons in the body making it hypersensitive and in turn magnesium helps calm the amygdala and the painful nerves. I believe 'the amygdala playing a big role in Fibro' is for the most part true as it is triggered and in a sense broken, in overdrive. Mind you, there is much research still that can go into this and either approve or disprove these theories. The brain is quite complicated and some doctors have stated that Fibro may be a result of the amygdala and the brain alone. This is the new thinking, mind you as I said, the brain and body should be treated together as one.

All in all, Fibro it seems is a physical AND emotional ailment.

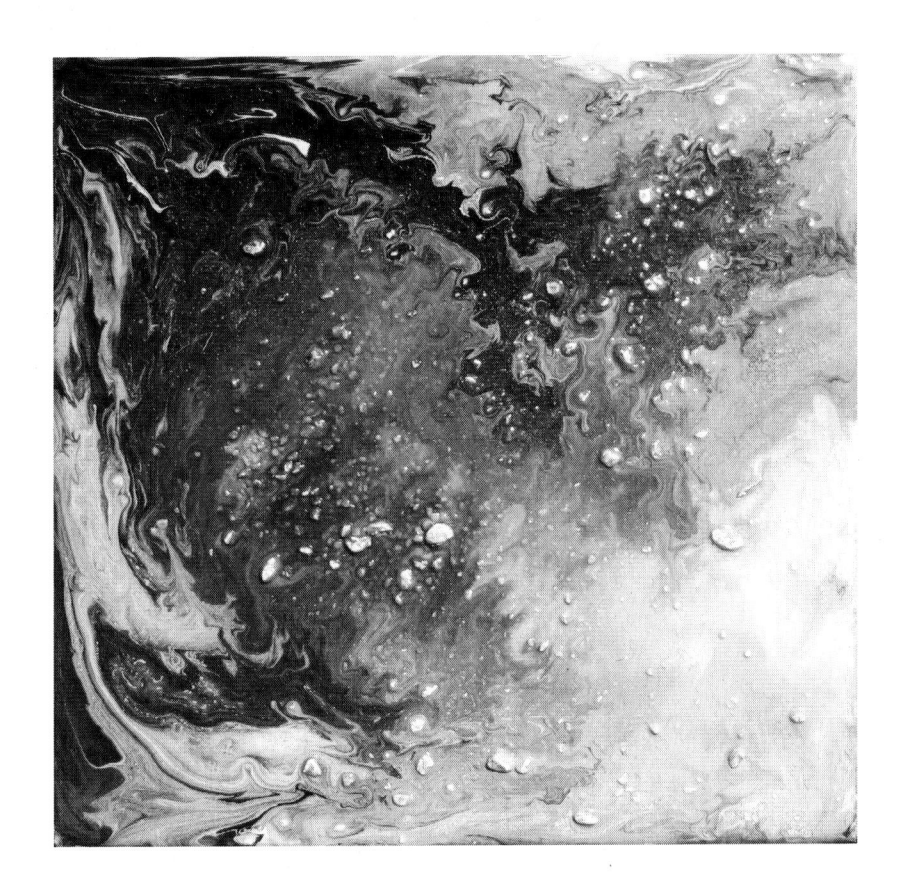

II. About Me and My Symptoms of Fibro, how long

I lay in bed, everything aches, my cat jumps on me- ouch, it hurts where his paws land on me- just the smallest touch to my skin and PAIN! The fatigue is so immense, too tired to get up and have a coffee or care for myself. The day consists of a shower, eat, a little cleaning and maybe one errand. Everything seems like a huge effort, even brushing my teeth. I get thru another day tho.
Mild antidepressants help a tad with the emotions and a bit of pain I understand. The odd Advil or Tylenol recommended by my doctor when symptoms kick in helps at times (but very toxic for liver ?). I spent months suffering and the weather playing havoc with my ailment. Up and down, like a see saw, one day good, next

few bad. Can't read because my brain doesn't seem to remember stuff, so it felt fruitless and dumb to try. No energy- depleted. Haven't worked but feel like I worked all day for days in a row with no rest and then got run over by a truck with all the pain. Brain fog, extreme pain, sensitivities, exhausted, anxious and feeling blue- no answers only questions- how does this happen, why, what can I do to help it (I am a problem solver, always).

Why do we know so little yet so many people suffer? Alot of women, esp supermoms, middle aged (but not always) may suffer. I feel like I need a cane to walk to get groceries or a wheelchair just to get around. I drive every where because I feel too tired to walk even a short distance, a block or two. People make fun of me and think I am lazy which adds to the destructiveness of the illness to the ego now. People don't believe you could feel or be sick because " you look so good". The invisible monster which overcomes ones body and eventually tries to take the soul.

After enough suffering and questions I decided to look into it myself and try to get better. I had no choice, no one was going to cure me and I had a big exam to write and start a new life and journey working in healthcare. So off I went to the local vitamin store. They at least believed but because almost all who worked there were so healthy they did not truly understand Fibro. They just knew alot of people suffered and no one knew answers- just guesses, kind of like mine. I bought a book on immune diseases, there was a blurb on Fibro- most about diet and vitamins and managing and understanding immunity, nothing cut and dry. Immunity seems to be key in Fibro. Is the body attacking itself- is CFS/Fibro really an autoimmune disease? Now what do I eat? Is it my diet? How do I lower my stress which seems to make it worse- vicious cycle- it causes more stress in your life which in turn makes it worse- real bad cycle. Yoga- certainly that will help with aches and pain and my mind. So I tried that. It seemed to work a little- help for the moment- tho meditation too was very important to calm the mind and remain optimistic. Hot baths. I tried that, that also helped relax me and was good for the body. Still no matter what I did it seemed like a drop in the bucket of solution and helped momentarily, not really big and long lasting.

My search continued- I tried some vitamins but again a drop. What is this and how does it come about? why me? why now? In the prime of my life yet. How can I get my health back?
Well one week thru a tough winter in Vancouver and here we are in January 2011. I felt the worst I had for one solid week- couldn't do anything to help. Just worse and worse. Pain, agony, my bones hurt thru and thru, couldn't move, could only lay in bed and almost cry (I believe I did). I thought for sure I was dying. This is ridiculous I thought. I am so young and should be healthy, I can't even care for myself and the pain and fatigue was becoming unbearable. I thought next week I will make out my 'will', surely I have some sort of cancer and am dying. This is not living?!

Depression was bad and I was isolated. No answers. Nobody. Well it was then that I took a huge dose of a mineral that was suppose to help a bit and it was like a darn miracle. It breathed life back into me. I regained my healthy feeling. I was optimistic.

Had I stumbled across "the cure" I thought ?! I felt so much better, the pain dissipated, energy came back. It took only a few hours to a couple days to feel all better (anyway a lot better!) and so with that here I give you my story , my success and findings, my gift to you. I may not be a doctor but it comes from the horses mouth, one who lived as you have and found a working solution (cheap too !!). The rest of the book should all make sense to you as it did me, as I finally pieced it all together, *"connected the dots"*. I feel literally cured from this mysterious modern day ailment called (labelled) "**Fibromyalgia**".

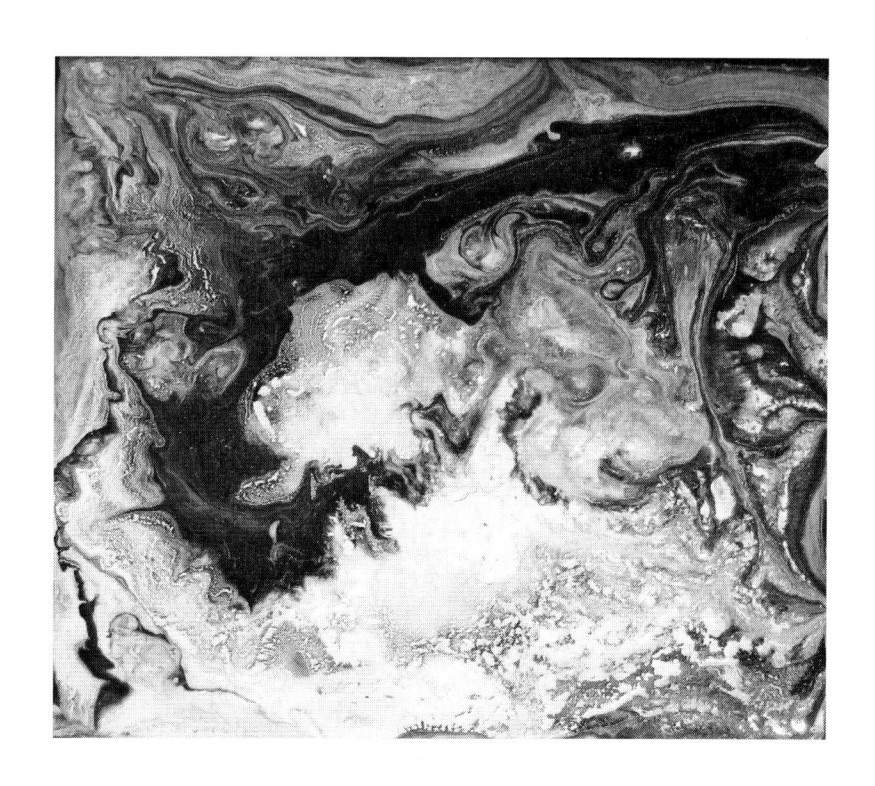

III. My Experimenting with fixes and the Magic Mineral Magnesium (Mg).

Anaemia commonly goes hand in hand with fibro and why it does I will get into later on.

Tried: Baths
yoga
diet- organic etc.
low dose Mg and vitamins (D & B's and A)
Carboxy acid (give energy)
muscle relaxants
pain relievers
Malic Acid mixture
Multivitamin
Ca/ Mg
antidepressants, tylenol, advil

Smoothies
Saw doctor (said I "did not look like typical fibro"
Sea vegetables (for hormones)
-Passion flower
-Udo's oil (PMS- irritability)
-adrenal therapy

... . all sound familiar?

What worked: Mg (2 grams (2000 mg) /day),
Vitamin D and
'Stress B vitamins'.

Magnesium (Mg) was taken 2 x 500 mg -am
1 x 500 mg-mid day
1 x 500 mg- at night (calms body and mind: helps with muscle aches/pains- sleep)

Vitamin D : 2 tablets (2000 IU)/day (helps depression/SADS)

Stress B Vitamin : 1 tablet/day
(help metabolism/**stress**/give energy)

*** Plus Adrenal Support ("Innate" brand with Ashwaghanda)

Magnesium (glycinate or bisglycinate) was the _MAGIC_ in high dose. High, High dose of 2-4 grams/day. **(help balance hormone levels, give energy and relieve pain) * (please see the section on the warning of too much Mg)**

How magnesium works I cover in a later chapter and why so important!

Now I do above (Mg+, D , B) (and)
- Ca+ and 'heavy metal removers' such as **Fulvic Acid**.
- 'epsom salt'(Mg) baths often using 1/2 - 1 cup /bath with sea salts (1/4 cup).
-meditation and mantra for mind (am and pm)
- Omega 3-6 -9 (need 3 esp) : high quality Fish oil.
- Udo's oil for mood - evens me. Or just Evening
- Primrose Oil (**EPO**) 500-1000mg/day- natural factors brand
-still antidepressants (low level)
- eat healthier, conscious diet, low sugar intake. (sensitivities lessening- almost all gone, no more light/noise sensitivity)
-Ashwaganda (replenish adrenals) & Rhodiola & Holy Basil
- replace or reduce coffee intake with green tea or Chai. (coffee= high cortisol.)
-try to exercise at least 30 minutes/day.
-green powder smoothie with whey protein powder in it.

and finally..-I have **REMOVED GLUTEN from my diet** and replaced with lots of fresh veg and fruit (and lots of water). (8 months ago quit- losing wt., no aches, better energy, clear brain – *whole chapter on in here of why so vital*)

I also do **Vegetable Powder** in Almond milk (OJ will spike blood sugar level), (add yogurt, banana and blend-smoothie) nearly EVERY DAY (get antioxidants, vitamins, enzymes and chlorophyll (Mg))

- very healthy choice and easy too.

I GIVE my full breakdown and 'Elimination' near the end of the book outlining in detail everything ! .....along with it's costs.

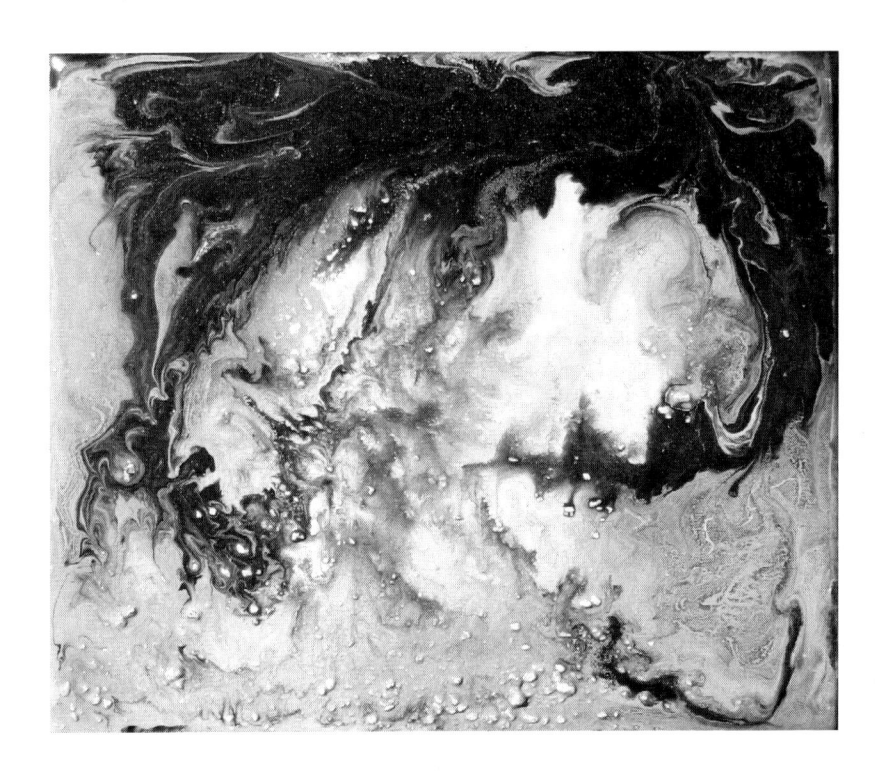

IV. FACTS ABOUT MAGNESIUM & CA++

What do I think causes Fibromyalgia, the root cause.....Well I have concluded thru my experience and experimenting and my wealth of knowledge of physiology which I draw upon, (mind you somewhat limited) that it is an issue with inflammation throughout the body and mind and due "in part" to alot of Calcium buildup in the tissues.

I use Magnesium to resolve Fibro, BUT Mg can cause severe diarrhoea, esp the Magnesium CITRATE.
(Magnesium exists in many combinations, magnesium glycinate, magnesium chloride, magnesium malate, etc. The form I most like and have less bowel problems with is the Magnesium (Bis)Glycinate, it seems most gentle while potent)
You see magnesium is very important to the body, it helps relax tissues and our minds. Calcium on the other hand has the ability

to contract. Calcium contracts, Magnesium relaxes, working in perfect balance at all times, in Yin Yang balance. When calcium is high, magnesium is low, and when magnesium is high, calcium is low, they work opposite.

I believe that due to high calcium in our environment (Dr.s in the past encouraged taking calcium), our lack of magnesium plus high calcium within our bodies in the form of bone, that these are all acting in imbalance and I will explain how.

Firstly, I'll explain Magnesium and our lack of it.
Magnesium is no longer coming from our water as it clogs the pipes (our water is now "softer"). In our soils in North America, Mg is depleted and the fertilizers and pesticides are high in Calcium. Also, our diet does not contain enough Mg in balance with Calcium as Calcium is found in our dairy products (now almond milk too!).
I could go into more detail about the lack but this is the basics. Plus our body is not absorbing enough Mg mainly due to a destroyed intestine which is due to gluten now. Also approx. 85% of Mg is absorbed in our gut by refined foods such as breads, etc , making it 'unavailable' to our bodies. Thusly, as we ingest Ca and not enough Mg, our balance is such that Ca high, Mg low. This means the Ca has to go somewhere and it finds it's way into our tissues and organs. Ca has the ability to contract and activate systems that work so the body, if too much Calcium will be in constant contraction and activation, thus wearing us out and stiffening everything. Too much Calcium is very bad for the heart and arteries, it makes them stiff.
Mg is important in over 300 enzymatic reactions in the body including (but not limited to) VERY important to the ***Krebs Cycle*** (energy- ATP). Mg will relax organs and muscles, helping energy to flow better. Mg relaxes arteries and actually lowers blood pressure.(Ca acts to harden arteries).
Mg is required to make **hormones** and Mg keeps Ca + in **fluid state** in the body so it does what it's suppose to. If low Mg, then

Ca is solid and goes to and gets trapped where it shouldn't be, like in tissues and organs (and arteries- esp the Aorta).

Calcium (Ca+):

When there is too high Calcium in the body the "Ca pumps" in cells are working harder to push it out of the cells, thus where it then goes is into the tissues, therefore alot of energy in the cells is thusly expended on the pumping and little else where energy is required in cells functioning properly. This is a very simple explanation in layman terms and when studied by researchers they will better detail it's aspects and how it works. <u>Ca is leached from the bones too when hormones are out of balance and just thru time.</u> This helps cause osteoporosis and weaken bones. This leached Ca is trapped in the tissues. When Mg is low in the body, it works that the Ca will thusly have to be high and if needed, then leached out of bone and into tissues, if this makes sense. Tissues and organs become stiff, hard and overworked.

This leads to fatigue and pain and I believe the inflammation works with it too as gluten which is over GMO'd now and not recognizable to our natural body as it is unnatural, the body launches an attack upon itself and the tissues & organs causing this inflammation. Inflammation causes much fatigue and pain, much like when you feel a flu, the body is launching an attack, it does not feel good and you feel very old and sick. Inflammation is most damaging to the blood vessels and leads to heart disease, CAD (coronary artery disease). How it works is that when inflammation damage occurs in vessels, the cholesterol in the body seeks these places out and tries to repair the scars and this forms plaques which may eventually break off due to high blood pressure one day and cause a stroke or heart attack. Mg keeps the vessels relaxed and open and healthy (not constricted like with Ca).
Lack of Mg I believe is a major cause of cancer, heart disease and Fibromyalgia, all on the rise since our soils are depleted, poisons

used (fertilizers), and our gluten (wheat) changed (altered) so drastically since the early 70's. It is very notable.

As we get older we lose more Mg, this is why we stiffen (skin) and wrinkle, it indicates what our organs are doing too. People who take enough Mg keep their skin soft, along with organs and they feel better and more relaxed (tend to rest and sleep better for repairing the body). When ones takes enough Mg, and it is not absorbed by refined foods, and makes it into cells, then the Ca will go down in concentration and is flushed out of the body or back into bones. The "calcium pumps" in cells will work easier and more efficient and everything relaxes and energy is now expended on other things the cells do. You feel energy (ATP and mitochondria working better)

Mg is very important to Mitochondria (the cells powerhouses for ATP) and it has been indicated in one article I read to be very effective in the treatment of Parkinson's disease as in Parkinson's the Mitochondria and their lack of functioning properly is a major feature and scientists are trying to create something to help make the Mitochondria (powerhouses of cells) work again. Just try alot of Mg I say. Inexpensive and might work!

Phosphorous also works in balance with Ca and Mg. From my reading, if too much phosphorous then Ca will leach from bones, not a good thing. The balance of all three is too technical to go into and I do not know enough about so I will not talk much about it. It is just common knowledge now about how Ca and Mg stay in balance together. Mg is quite an amazing mineral if you read about it and all the diseases it can cure from Parkinson's and Arthritis to Mental Illness (anxiety esp). Where other countries are not as deficient in Mg as us, they show less disease, especially heart disease. Australia in contrast, has very soft water (low Mg, mineral content) and is #1 in Heart Disease (CAD) in the world. So in conclusion of this chapter, it is logical to suggest that the buildup of Ca in tissues (body) and lack of Mg along with inflammation due to gluten (diet) stands to be the reason for so much pain and fatigue experienced by people with Fibromyalgia (along with all the other symptoms). I do not go into what too much Ca does to the brain because I think it is largely unknown but it may cause some plaque formation along with inflammation (gluten) and the Ca keeps the mind on high alert, thus the sensitivities, stress, irritability, brain fog and depression (and regularly insomnia). I did read when we are stressed (ie. Over sensitive) that it damages the DNA in our brain, thus the grey hair with it. Stress helps cause mental illnesses (ie. Anxiety, depression, nervous breakdowns).

And it has been discussed in wheat belly how gluten affects even psychosis and hallucinations.

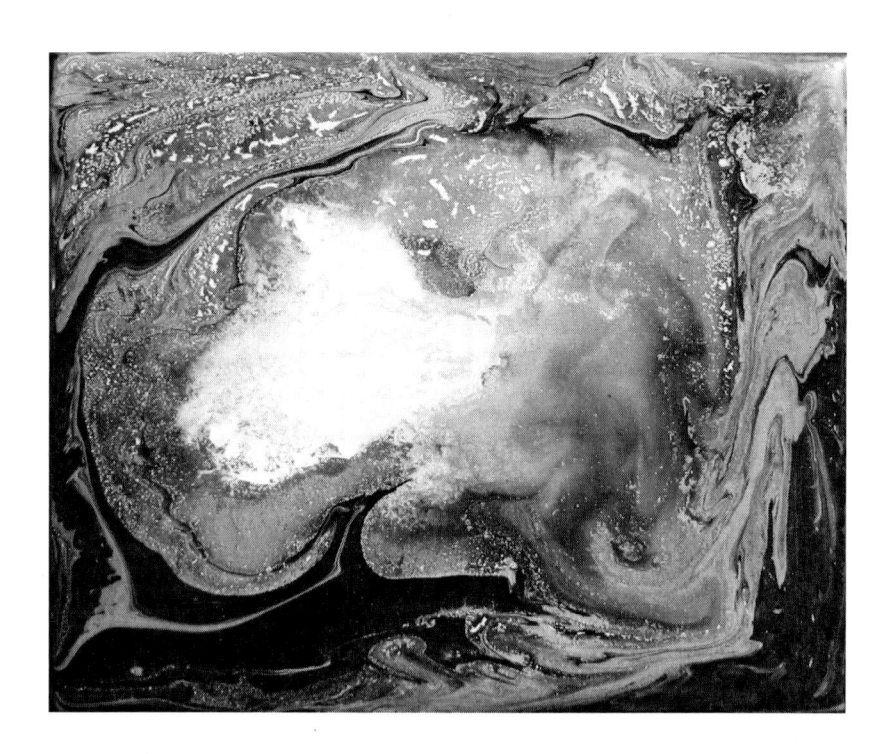

V. WHY More Women Affected Than Men

Why more women than men are affected is simply about :

(1) ***Estrogen*** and ***hormonal imbalances***.
More Testosterone in men = less cortisol (*stress hormone*)

There is also a difference in (2) our ***brain structure*** and how we process info, emotions and stress (too detailed for here, just know that women's brains are more active and emotional than men's and thus probably more prone to stress) I talk about the brain in random related topics.

There is also the topic of (3) ***adrenal burnout*** because women have less testosterone, we have more, higher cortisol, the stress hormone. Too much pumping out of cortisol burns the adrenals out (I cover in detail later here).

Estrogen and Hormonal Imbalances:
1. **Estrogen** has an effect on Calcium (Ca) in the body which can be better explained by a scientist per say, so I will not go into grave detail here as is unnecessary to understand it exactly, just that Estrogen and Calcium work in unisance. If high Estrogen, high Ca- If low Estrogen, low Ca. *(Ca will come from bones (leached) to balance off low Mg)*

Thus, Low Mg = High Ca = High Estrogen (the equation)
and, **High Estrogen = High Ca = Low Mg = Fibromyalgia**

Through my reading I have found that with Estrogen as it goes up, so does Ca in the body. As we lose Estrogen, say in menopause, then Ca goes down in the body, that is why doctors suggest women supplement with Ca/Mg vitamins, so that Ca will not leach from bones to make up for it and thusly encourage osteoporosis. So you may say then if Estrogen goes down and thusly Ca as women age, then shouldn't Fibromyalgia not exist in older women, as I have implied it exists due to high Ca (high estrogen)?

Well here is an explanation for that:
There exists in our environment alot and I mean alot more Estrogen then ever before and we get it into our bodies. For instance, as ridiculous as this sounds it is even on our paper and when we touch paper (like receipts) our bodies can absorb it (I am still looking for some evidence of this tho). There are alot of whats called 'Phyto-Estrogens' now too which tend to mimic Estrogen. So if we do take in alot more Estrogen from our environment it will lead to more Ca, thus more health problems as earlier discussed.

If Estrogen is low, then the Ca is low (automatic). If our Mg is low (deficient due to environment and diet) our Ca needs to thusly increase (as it is low), thus the body then grabs it from bones to 'up' the Ca level.(thus then leached from our bones into tissues).

We need both Mg and Ca for good strong bones (neither leached).

Thusly again, our Mg is low in our bodies (diet, as we age, etc) , then Ca needs to be high (the body's own balancing) and this Ca then comes mainly from bones as it has to come from somewhere (bones are an immediate and reliable source for the body). If we supplement Ca without Mg it leads to problems with imbalance and too much Ca stresses the body.

When supplementing with Ca I think scientists and doctors are unclear about how much goes into bones and how much stays in tissues. Mg apparently works in the body to liquify Calcium so Ca can be absorbed by the bones but if not liquid state, Ca will collect where it is not suppose to, like say tissues and vessels.

I know alot of people who supplement with Ca when they should really be supplementing with Mg and pushing Ca back into the bones (out of tissues) where it belongs and not in the tissues. *Ca in tissues causes contraction and stiffening. People age and become very rigid due to this lack of Mg, and they "lose" it in the brain!*

ESTROGEN AND THE BRAIN:

2. Brain structure
As I mentioned in the beginning of this chapter, women's brains are fundamentally different then men's. Their size and structure differ. Probably due to estrogen forming the brain structure in babies. Men have alot of grey matter which is the outer edges of the brain and when they process incoming information it stays mainly in these areas when they react and think. Women on the other hand, process incoming information differently as when the info comes in, it hits the grey matter first then bounces all around the brain sending signals to all the other parts of the brain, they essentially `think more` about things and it gets sent to their

emotional centres wherein they tend to react and thusly talk alot. This is why men can easily turn off and women easily turn on. On brain scans of each sex, these differences show up and are proven by how the brain lights up in different areas of the brain when stimulated and how active it all is. In a mans scan there is not much activity thus not alot of areas light up except for the surrounding grey matter. In a women's scan however the whole brain is lite up when getting info and processing it, it bounces from the grey matter to the limbic system (emotions) and to the pre-frontal cortex (reasoning) where they try to reason everything. So there you go, proof women do over think and overreact while men are cool, logical and laid back. Men always thought it was a hormonal thing but now it`s proven it is a anatomical-nervous system brain thing.

Being Gay: "...... is being gay a brain issue?"
I am going to go out on a limb and suggest that being gay is rooted in an organ, the brain. I believe our hormones form our brain structure depending on how much of each Estrogen and Testosterone are produced and this then affects which sex we are most attracted to. So I believe like many that we are born this way. Having more Estrogen seems drawn to and attracted to the look of a man and having more Testosterone is attracted to the look of a woman. Maybe pheromones and hormones interacting? It may show physically different (our sex organs) but it is the brain and how it functions that matters in who we better relate to. Thus, Gay men will tend to be more emotional than straight men as they will tend to have more estrogen than them. And Gay women will likely have more testosterone than a straight female, thus be more calm. I would then conclude that gay men are more likely to end up having fibromyalgia as they react different to stress (more like a women) and over think things due to the structure of the brain and the present hormones that are produced. (hope I am not stepping on any toes!)

How does brain structure affect Fibro you ask, well **stress plays a key role in Fibro** as all who deal with it are aware and when the brain over processes info in the brain like a women's does then this releases and causes more stress to occur (activates the fight or flight system) and also impacts all their relationships, work or home alike, and this induces unnecessary stress, making Fibro worse. And it remains a viscous cycle of when you add stress, the pain and fatigue increases and this then causes more stress in ``feeling worse`` and so it goes, around and around. *I cover a section later on `reacting`.* Just being too emotional is in itself stressful for all. This stress can help burn out the adrenals. Always best to just remain calm and cool.

Estrogen and Soy :

Soy Protein or Soy Protein Isolate causes an increase in Estrogen in the body as the core of the soybean is loaded with Estrogen and this is what the Soy Protein is, all the good outer stuff is stripped away. If you want a good source of soy make sure the label reads, "ground whole soy" in either soy milks or other products. Good soy to have is Miso, Tempeh or Natto (all Asian), all fermented and whole sources, very good for you as it will contain the omega3's and healthy carbs and actually help balance the hormone levels. (Aside: Lentils and hemp are good sources of protein for a person.)

As a caution Soy is not good to have if you are on thyroid medication (ie. synthroid) as it interrupts it's proper function. Thus, Soy increases Estrogen, which increases Ca and increases Fibro. I tend to believe that the abundance of "Stripped Soy" is a problem in Fibro (I do almond milk myself) .

HORMONES

Hormonal imbalances causes all sorts of problems with the body from thyroid, metabolism to brain imbalances (namely PMS - mood, irritability). So the fact that we must better balance our hormones is very important (thru diet mainly) and I think more so for women than for men at least right now. We have really messed with hormones in our environment and food, say like all the hormones farmers feed their animals, this goes into our bodies too. Chicken, for instance is really bad for extra hormone content as farmers try to grow them quickly.
People with Fibro often have a severe hormonal imbalance (irritability and sensitivity).

One thing I find absolutely brilliant at helping with 'hormone balance and MOOD' is **Evening Primrose Oil (EPO**), it is a **miracle PMS buster**! Has saved my life. Is definitely "natures mood stabilizer" and should be tried by anyone who wants to settle down their irritability level and thus improve all the relationships in their life and mostly to be who you really are and not your mood!
I Most favour the brand Omega/Natural factors- ULTRA PRIM

(If I could patent it, I would be rich and trust me someone will try to make it a drug and patent it as a mood stabilizer) Just like the drug "Lyrica" has Mg in it and helps Fibro.

Testosterone in Men:

Men naturally have more testosterone than women and science has proven that with **more testosterone, one has less cortisol.** Cortisol is relative to the adrenals and it is partly due to adrenal burnout that Fibro exists. With high cortisol output, it taxes the adrenals and wears them out = adrenal burnout = Fibro (women)

3. ADRENAL BURNOUT & Hormones:

Adrenal burnout is also referred to as "adrenal fatigue" and this is when the adrenals produce less than adequate cortisol for the body. Many things lead to burnout or fatigue as all the 'stressors' in our lives add up and impact our minds and bodies, positive or negative, either all at once or chronically over time. When stress occurs, the body gets a fight or flight signal and this causes the hypothalamus to signal the pituitary to signal the adrenals to then release cortisol. The cortisol is sent out to basically "protect the cells under this stress". Stressors can be any I listed under stress in this book in a later chapter, including nutritional (dietary). The result of adrenal burnout is mainly fatigue. Second is foggy brain.

CORTISOL:

A healthy adrenal gland (we have two, each sit on top of each kidney) will excrete cortisol when signalled by the brain, it is a cascade of steps and actions to produce cortisol.
Cortisol helps PROTECT the cells of the body and keep them healthy. It has an anti-inflammatory response too and helps regulate insulin. We normally release the most cortisol at around 8 am, this wakes us up, it fluctuates throughout the day depending on eating and stressors. Lowest between midnight and 4 am for most people (when we sleep). If the body does not release enough cortisol throughout the day we feel sluggish and tired, it gives us the "umph" we need to get things done and stay awake. So some cortisol is healthy and good, too much disastrous.

Too much stress or 'trauma' can lead to the over release of cortisol (too much that overwhelms the system) and this becomes damaging. When one gets stressed either over time or in a short burst this can lead to over action of the adrenals and they burnout. There are a few good books on this topic so I don't really go into it, but briefly as it could be a book on it's own, I am just pointing to adrenal burnout as a contributing cause of Fibro (as I am sure alot of people with Fibro feel adrenal burnout and this could help explain why people who endure extreme trauma in their lives can become susceptible to Fibro.)

Things to help if you have Adrenal burnout:
    Vit C, (helps neutralize cortisol- very key one)
    Vit E
 and Vit B,
    Mg and trace minerals, (kelp - excellent source of Mg)
 * **Herbs** : Ashwaghanda, Ginseng, Holy Basil, Rhodiola

Sources of Mg are brown rice, beans, nuts and seeds as well as the leafy greens and sea vegetables like Kelp (best source of Mg). Sea vegetables like kelp have chlorophyll in them (chlorophyll=Mg). Mg assists with the cortisol cascade and in energy production. Mg is responsible as I have previously mentioned in important enzymes and for energy (ATP- Krebs cycle).

If adrenals burn out and are exhausted, often women with too much stress hormone have belly fat. This belly fat gives off (makes) hormones adding to imbalance (estrones). Then the thyroid takes the next beating as hormones are thrown out of balance and can thus malfunction (affect mood swings). Hypothyroidism and obesity is on the rise and yes more common in women than in men. Added stress (computers- always plugged in) and coffee nowadays makes our adrenals burn out quicker. Our adrenals burning out is why staryucks and spanks are multimillionaires. Stimulant needed (coffee) as tired, and now chubby (spandex needed).

Coffee can make one hypoglycemic as well and hypoglycemia leads to moodiness, maybe partly why since staryucks we have gotten moodier as a nation? (more stressed and unhealthy)

Why more women than men prone to adrenal burnout:

Approximately 6:1 or 9:1 women to men get Fibro. (varies). It varies because I believe men are under diagnosed as well as the difference in Hormones and brains. Testosterone levels are in balance with cortisol levels in the body such that when testosterone is high, cortisol is low. And when testosterone is low, cortisol is high! So this partly explains the male/female difference and ratio as women have much less testosterone in their bodies than men do, thus their cortisol levels will be higher. This leads to adrenal burnout and affect on the brain as far as cortisol having the fight or flight response. Makes good sense. It has been explained that the amygdala in the centre of the brain which directs the fight or flight response plays a major role in Fibro. I don't believe it's all the brain (as some now attest it is solely the brain), but rather a physical and emotional role together acting. They are deeply linked together, one affects the other just as a high emotional state such as anxiety can cause increased Blood Pressure in people, a physiological phenomenon. The above is why I believe you must support your adrenals and thus try to control your cortisol levels to get a grip on Fibro as well as work on the physical part; healing your gut and getting vital nutrients, vitamins, minerals, H2O and rest.

Mg helps calm the mind and I believe the Amygdala. It will help settle the fight or flight response and tone down anxiety, thus work on mental and physical as you heal your adrenals. But you must be able to absorb it! (may need injections?).

I believe Mg works directly on the hyperactive Amygdala (on high alert fight or flight) to calm it. (thus calm the brain).

One of my friends recently took Kelp for her thyroid for energy and to her surprise it worked, she likely has adrenal burnout too. I believe if you burn out the adrenals, the thyroid is next as adrenals play an important role in hormone regulation as well. The thyroid plays a vital role in hormone regulation. All connected. I know with me I feel my adrenals have been burnt out

for about 20 years and I have been sold so many remedies to help it over that time. The best I have come across is a mix of herbs including ashwaganda (the innate brand) and taking Mg. When you think about it if we take Mg, it calms the mind and helps us deal with stress thus, less triggering of the fight or flight response and giving the adrenals a rest, to recover.
I fully believe the adrenals have the ability to recover and regain their proper and full function if given what they need to heal and like with us, they need assistance (dietary) and a rest (low stress/proper sleep). It will take time I believe to regain the adrenals. I believe the body has an amazing ability to recover over most anything, even the brain can recover and that is largely the nervous system which is toughest to regain. The body is really a phenomenal machine, always working to be it's best and work optimally if given the proper crutches.

There is alot more to cover for adrenal burnout but instead there are some fabulous books out there if you want to know more, I just describe here basically it's role & influence in fibromyalgia. I think personally it makes alot of sense.

I believe also the core of all disease is in our DIET (plus genetic predisposition) and what we put into our bodies to help it function, just like you would a machine you rely on to function optimally. What you put into your brain is equally important too and I have run across some studies that state that thinking negatively actually does have a biological impact on the body (in a negative way, destroying it). **We have a physiological response to negative thoughts.**

What we are fed today both in diet and TV ties into alot of our modern day diseases, even news is so dramatic and for the most part always so negative. I try to stay away from stressful horror stories or movies, violence and alot of negative news, I just get enough so I don't have my head in the sand. I watch reality based stories that tend to be inspirational, motivating and happy. This is what I feed my head. Nutritionally I try to eat the best I can without being perfect as I am about 90% gluten free, not 100%, I think it is too much pressure with all that is around to be 100% free.

I take vitamins I need for myself and the trace minerals which can be particularly in sea salt. It is really ones responsibility to be their own best source and doctor nowadays. Keep a journal and use trial and error method as I did. The internet if used properly and knowingly can be an excellent source for **information and stories from others.**

HELPS ADRENALS AND STRESS HORMONES:
Ashwaganda and B vitamins, Holy Basil and Rhodiola also.

1. <u>Ashwaganda (Indian Ginseng)</u>- helps balance stress hormones, adrenalin in body. Nourishes and heals the adrenals. ('Innate- adrenal response', is a whole food and a good brand to try- has everything you need in it- I get mine from Finlandia)

2. <u>B vitamins</u>- help deal with stress (research says)- needed to calm system. Important in fibromyalgia- a Multi- B.

3. <u>Holy Basil and Rhodiola</u>- Help calm nerves and body too. Mellows people out. (ask nutritionist about).

4. <u>Thyrosmart and kelp</u> - nourishes the thyroid. regain some balance of hormones: has L-tyrosine (selenium also needed for thyroid)

5. <u>Vitamin D</u>- need enough Mg in body to absorb this, helps with SADS, which affects stress levels if your mood gets low.

If adrenals burn out and are exhausted, often women with too much stress hormones have belly fat - then thyroid takes the next beating and can malfunction. Hypothyroid on the rise- obesity.

FIBROSUCCESS

Computers are actually added stress and all the coffee nowadays makes our adrenals burn out quicker.

6.   <u>Vitamin C</u> - neutralizes cortisol (calming antioxidant) (good for skin-collagen)

7.   **<u>L-Theanine</u>**- calms the mind and nerves. **Works wonders!** (derivative of green tea)

<u>Conclusion of Adrenal Burnout and Women</u>:

So in a nutshell, I believe ones high cortisol levels (due mainly to stress) burns out your adrenals which affect your hormones and thyroid functioning (hormones, metabolism, energy) The imbalanced **hormones intimately connected to the brain**, affects the brains functioning physically and emotionally (irritability, irrational thoughts or reasoning, indecision) and this affects the thought processes as one feels they cannot control their thoughts which then affect the body in every physical way. So one needs to stop the cortisol, heal the adrenals, calm the mind and work on positive thinking.
Usually people with Fibro will drive others absolutely nuts, people lose their patience, it is because their mind is so scrambled up. They are irritable and thus irritate others, this makes relationships so very difficult. They also seem very needy and self focused and self absorbed, this due to the brain and illness taking over. They cannot think outside the illness. It gets exhausting for all.

Get a grip on your stress and your thoughts at the same time, meditate, think happy thoughts continuously and take Mg and L-theanine to calm the firing of the neurons in the brain which causes this irritability and negativity and indecision. I am sure if scientists scanned the brains of Fibro people and compared to regular people, they'd find in Fibro patients the Pre-frontal cortex light up more often (due to hormone imbalances- like PMS symptoms).

Scientists are only now beginning to be aware of how intimately hormones are connected to the brain and thus the ensuing importance of this.

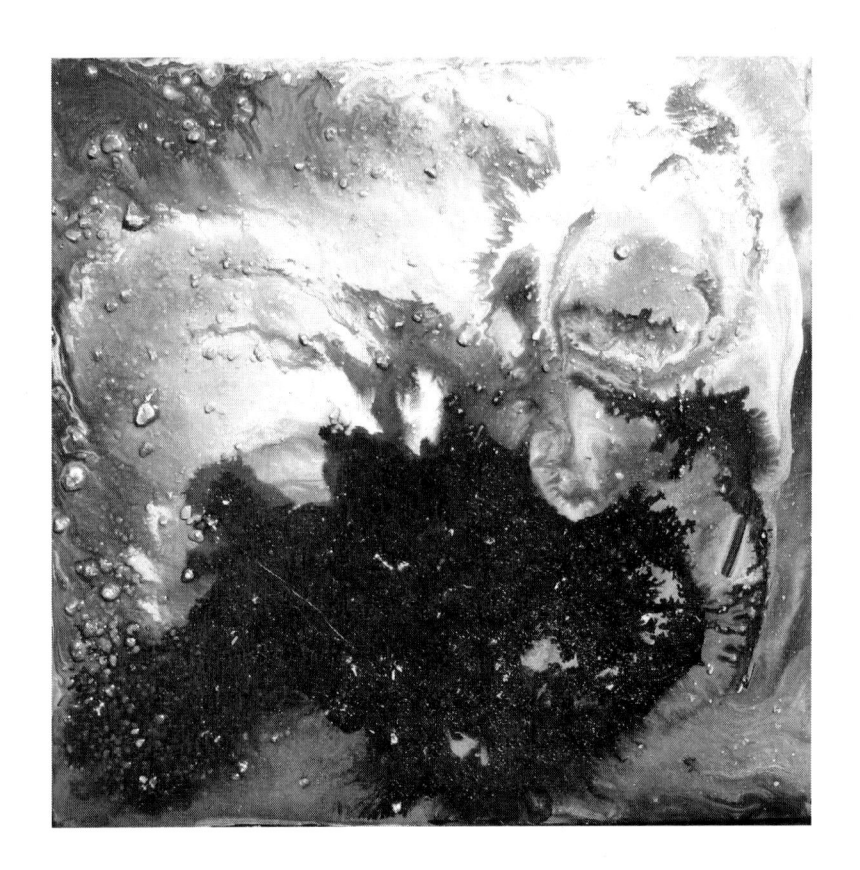

VI. Why Mg works, in my opinion. & other diseases Mg can help with.

Mg is crucial to more than 300 bodily functions- many of which give you <u>energy</u>.

some Mg containing foods are:
-chocolate (mainly dark)
-bananas
-kidney beans
-black beans
-whole wheat bread (will have gluten)
-brown rice
-lentils
-oatmeal (may have gluten?)

-quinoa
- raisan Bran (may have gluten)
- spinach
- shredded wheat (gluten)
(I cover more later)

need approx. 5 servings/day

FACT: 3/4 of Americans are Mg deficient – called
"Hypomagnesia".

-are you irritable, tired, weak? if so read on,

covered:
1. How Mg works, in my opinion
2. How it can help; food sources
3. Other diseases Mg can help with
4. Warnings of too much Mg

Magnesium is the 4 th most abundant mineral in the body and involved in more than 300 biochemical reactions. Magnesium is required for good Vitamin B & Vit D absorption. Magnesium makes up a good portion of bones and teeth, as Ca acts like a chalk and Mg acts like the superglue. Both are needed for mineralization.

In today's world we are told to take Ca+ supplements and we get alot already from our food sources. Mg is low in today's soils and has been depleted from the soils and water sources in the past 50 years or so. Mg tends to clog the city pipes so it is found in only small amounts in city water. Ca+ is found in higher amounts as it is in fertilizers, etc. Thus we are getting plentiful Ca+ while falling short of Mg.

Mg, Ca and Phosphorous (Ph) all exist in a seesaw balance in the body.

When Ca is high, Mg is low (and visa-versa) and when phosphorous is high both Ca and Mg are low. Phosphorous pushes Ca and Mg into bones and causes mineralization to occur. All are required in the body but one must be aware of the amounts one is getting or exposed to both in diet and supplement, and realize how they affect each other. It has been determined that the average person gets 1000 mg Ca+ in the daily diet alone. When one supplements Ca+ in the body, then Mg will go down and get flushed out.

It works sort of like this:

Ca+ high= Mg low
Ca+ low= Mg high
Ph high= Ca+ low, Mg low
Ph low= Ca+ high, Mg high

Mg and Ca are in a seesaw relationship and together they exist in another seesaw relationship with phosphorous.

Ca works to contract muscles and in abundance will collect in organs, joints and tissues and too much can cause stiffness in organs and joints. As women age the Ca gets leached from the bones this probably due to low Mg. A person needs high Ca in the blood to balance the seesaw and if Ca is not in the diet, it will leach out of the bones, to balance. Maybe, just maybe with menopause (age) we lose Mg and this makes Ca come out of bones. Therefore the equation and seesaw of Low Mg = High Ca. We must add more Mg so this shifts to high Mg= Low Ca and keeps Ca in the bones where it belongs.

Magnesium is vital to energy production (ATP) and explains alot in the realm of fatigue if we get too little. As stated above three quarters of Americans are Mg deficient. Mitochondria are the energy powerhouses of cells, they produce what is called ATP (Adenosine Tri-Phosphate).

Without Mitochondria we don't produce energy (ATP).

Mg and Mitochondria rely on each other. A cell (muscle) contracts by pushing Ca+ out of the cell, if too much Ca in tissue and extra cellular fluid, this exhausts the cell as it cannot pump Ca+ out and this uses up vital energy reserves (lowered ATP) ATP is required to do the pumping. Thus, one will feel fatigued. When we add Mg, this lowers Ca in surrounding extracellular fluid and thus Ca can more easily be pushed out of the cell and cause a contraction (muscle movement say). If too much Ca - contraction then exists and is exhausting. Magnesium causes muscles to relax and is a good sleep aid as it helps the brain relax and be calm.

In a crisis, it is beneficial to take a high dose of Mg to calm the brain down. Thus Mg and Ca work opposite each other, Ca to contract muscle, Mg to relax. Both are required. It is just that due to our depleted soils and food sources of Mg that we get too little and our Ca intake being more increased, puts it way out of balance :

High Ca=low Mg= Contraction= No Energy, stiff, rigid, & old

I believe this imbalance is the number one cause of aging in people.

I will not go into greater chemical detail as it is not so important, one can research it if curious, I have just laid out the basics and summary. I am sure a biochemist would know alot more than I, even tho I studied some.
Thus this is all why I strongly believe Fibro is due to Ca in the connective tissues and organs, and causing Pain and cramping and lack of energy in the body (fatigue). Makes good sense does it not?

Calcium and Aging: (Ca+ & CAD)

Ca ages us too. Mg is like a youth drug, makes us soft and flexible while Ca makes us all stiff, rigid and inflexible. Ca gives us tough, wrinkled skin too. (so does stress). Is this why at the same age men often look younger than women?: Stress, Cortisol? Too much Ca leads to cardiovascular problems as it helps cause arteriosclerosis. Ca collects in arteries as plaques, makes arteries less flexible and rather hard and stiff. This rigidity and stiffness of arteries contributes to high blood pressure and also arteries may rupture due to stress on them where too much Ca exists. I also believe that too much Ca can lead to stiffness of the heart but then that is just my opinion. Thus, it is very probable and researched that Mg relaxes arteries, makes them soft and flexible and in doing so, helps reduce blood pressure. Mg is an easy solution to high BP vs. drugs which often result in bad side effects.

Ca is also not good for the heart muscle and can instigate heart attacks. Remember it causes contraction of muscles and the heart is a muscle. High Ca can cause CAD (Coronary artery disease). We need a healthy balance of Ca and Mg for the heart to function properly. Mg helps with lowering cholesterol and fats as well. Mg helps open arteries, Ca closes them. I have also tried Arginine for healthy arteries, this is suppose to be good and work too. Helps open arteries and keep soft too.

MAGNESIUM SOURCES:
Mg is low nowadays as 85% of Mg is lost when flour is refined, bleached and processed (they remove the germ and bran). Therefore it's not in our grains anymore. As well, approx. 80% of Mg ingested is 'not absorbed' when we consume gluten and wheat in our diet.

Wheat and gluten are the 'go to' nowadays. It seems it is everywhere, in everything.

So if we are not getting enough Mg here are some good food sources to look out for if you want a good balance :

FOOD SOURCES OF Mg:
Almonds, cashews
Spinach
 Soybeans
Nuts, Peanuts
Wheat Bran
Peanut butter
Potato baked with skin
Black-eye peas
Pinto Beans
Rice, Brown, black
Lentils
Kidney beans
Chocolate milk
Banana
Yogurt
Milk chocolate
Milk
Raisins
Halibut
Whole wheat bread (is not bleached)
Avocado
Chocolate Pudding
eggs (I am not sure ?)
Buckwheat
Baking cottonseed
Chocolate (oh did I already say that)
Tofu
Tea
Collard greens and parsley
soybean flour
Beets
Kale

Brocolli
Anything green with chlorophyll

Basically, it is in whole grains, dark green leafy vegetables (chlorophyll) and fish such as halibut and Cod, Beans and legumes (soybeans, lentils, peanuts) and nuts. Alot of things organic are good too as the soil hopefully is better and a good source. I believe this is what helps some Fibro patients who eat organic, their sensitivities will go down due to the possible Mg that exists within their organic diets.

OTHER DISEASES Mg HELPS:

Basically Mg is calming and relaxing and adds energy while assisting Musculo-skeletal issues and aiding the heart.
It impacts the brain a great deal, alot more then most scientists I think even realize or have studied. **Mg affects the body physically and mentally.**

Mg helps with:
Sleep(insomnia), **Parkinson's***(the mitochondria- ATP), Diabetes, ED (erectile dysfunction), Alzheimers- senility,* **Mental Illness**, **Anxiety**, *Migraines, Rheumatoid Arthritis, maybe MS, etc.*

Sleep (insomnia) and Mg
Mg is often a sleep aid. It helps calm and relax the mind probably working on the Amygdala and stress levels. Take half hour before bed to sleep.
(Tart Cherry Juice works too as it contains melatonin which helps sleep. Take one 7oz glass one hour before bed, or eat a handful dried.)

Mg has been shown to help with Depression, Mental Illness and Anxiety, all symptoms of Fibro.

SUPPLIES OF Mg:

Magnesium exists in many combinations, magnesium glycinate, magnesium chloride, magnesium citrate (will give you the runs) etc., the form I most like and have less bowel problems with is the 'Magnesium Glycinate', it seems most gentle while potent. You can take alot of it in that form without the diarrhoea I found for myself, you may too.(and I am sensitive)
(I buy mine at FINLANDIA, Vancouver BC Canada)

how much to take etc.

2 grams for approx. 2 weeks then 1 gram for few months til better then 500 mg/day (maintenance, just when feel low, cramps or achey).
I hardly take at all anymore tho I will start taking a maintenance level soon again after I know how Gluten Elimination is affecting Fibro.

Important:

WARNING OF TAKING TOO MUCH Mg

Mg supplementation should be **AVOIDED with severe kidney problems** (severe renal insufficiency when on dialysis) and also with Myasthenia Gravis. (or too low of blood pressure)

Use caution if you have severe adrenal weakness or low blood pressure. If one consumes too much Mg, this can cause muscle weakness, if this occurs just use more calcium temporarily to relieve. Signs and symptoms of too much Mg (hypermagnesia) can be similar to magnesium deficiency and include:

changes in mental status, diarrhoea (dehydration), nausea,

appetite loss, muscle weakness, difficulty breathing, extremely low blood pressure, dizziness, and irregular heartbeat.

Just because your body rids Mg as it is water soluble, does not mean that excessive amounts over time cannot be somewhat harmful, if you feel you are encountering a problem please seek medical attention or take the high doses of Mg UNDER the care of a Professional who can monitor any side effects of high dose Mg.

Just be aware that most doctors, especially Western won't be agreeable with this method and may fight you on it because of either lack of knowledge or the safety concerns mentioned above pending your individual situation or case. If they truly fight you on it and you feel strongly about trying it, I suggest to just try a high dose for 'maybe one week only' and see if you notice a difference (take with lots of water).

Just please be aware of how you feel and any negative changes as everyone reacts differently and just because I did not have problems doesn't mean you won't necessarily. Just because it is natural does not mean it cannot be toxic to the body or not cause problems. Take this with caution.

Journal how you feel if you like and show your doctor. I am rather against high doses for a prolonged period of time like more than 3- 6 months.

The best is to try to decrease the Ca levels in your tissues and use a maintenance level of Mg or a balance of Mg and Ca long term.

If you feel you have a problem due to high Mg, please seek medical attention for help, right away.

FIBROSUCCESS

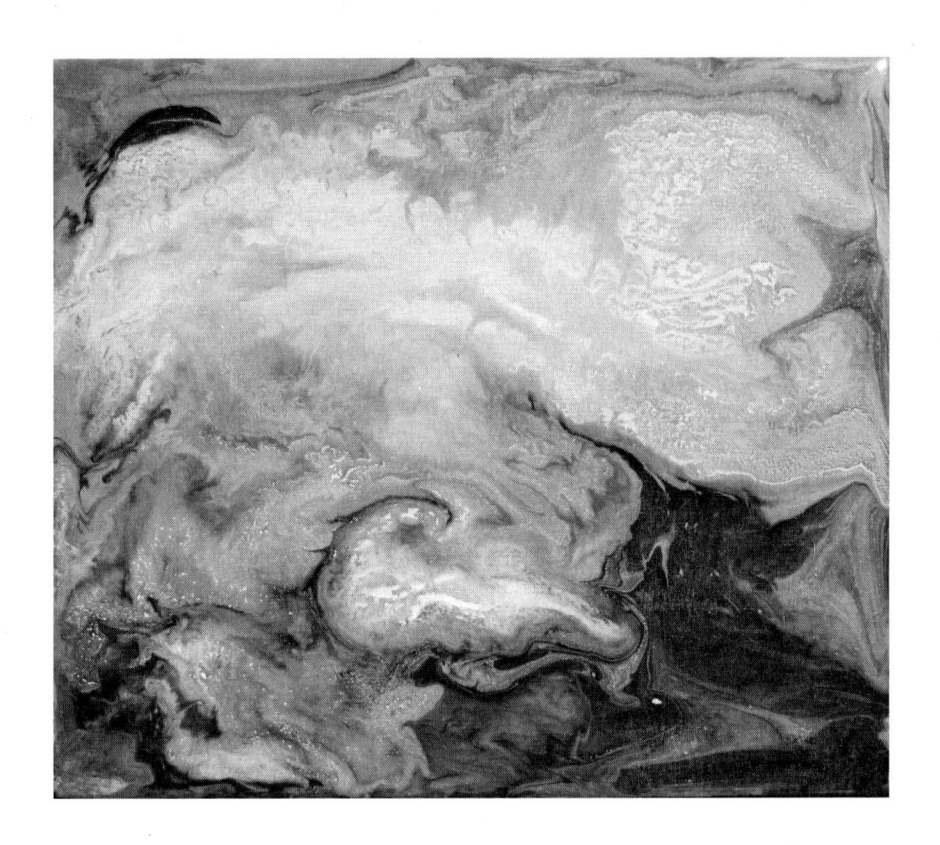

VII. GLUTEN:
(Inflammation- gluten riddance)

"THE GLUTEN CONNECTION"

Let me discuss Gluten a little, just basically.

Gluten Intolerant, Gluten Sensitive : are you sensitive to gluten?

GLUTEN IS: Wheat, Barley and Rye (yes whole grain bread!)
 A bit about gluten: is a wheat, rye or barley grain found most often in bread products or soups (thickeners) or dressings. Your gut will react to it if it cannot process it. Over 25,000 different strains are produced now in North America (used to be about 2 in early 1900's), it is GMO'd (genetically modified

organism) way too much that it causes health problems for people. Wheat used to be a four foot long flowing branch of wheat which is now reduced and changed to something that is about one foot in height and resembles a tough bush. They have made it so that it is more disease resistant, higher yielding for farmers and has helped assist with world hunger. When gluten is not processed by the body properly and rather causes a reaction, it can thus attack the body and cause inflammation.

Common outcomes (results) of Gluten Sensitivity (GS) are:

-depression/ anxiety/ neurological problems
-obesity (tummy)
-heart disease (inflammation of arteries; plaques)
-hormone imbalance
-diabetes (also tummy and high blood sugar levels)
-rashes
-hair loss

Some classic symptoms of GS are:

:fatigue
:throw up/diarrhoea/constipation
:bloating/gas
:cloudy thinking (brain fog)
:IBS (irritable bowel syndrome)- acid reflux like symptoms
:aches and pains (due to inflamed joints)
:mood swings (hormone imbalance)
:CFS/Fibro like symptoms

Dr. Oz had a self test for people with GS not too long ago on his show, it included these issues:
> **digestive**- bloat/gas
> IBS acid reflux
> diarrhoea/constipation

neurological- headaches/migraines
-joint aches and pains
-brain fog
hormonal - depression/ anxiety
-chronic fatigue
-chronic eczema and acne

(to the best of my memory)......if you had 4 or more of these symptoms you likely have a problem with gluten.
Approx. 10-20% of people are GS (Gluten sensitive) (maybe higher like 30%).

Celiac disease (completely intolerant to gluten) is about 1% of the population, most statistics say.
In Celiacs, The antibodies produced cause intestinal damage. (found with blood test)

With gluten sensitivity all tests are negative, there is a high percentage who are, approx. 20 million or 1/10 adults (or 10% and this estimate is on the low end).

If your doctor cannot help diagnose a problem then try getting gluten OUT of your diet. Easy to do. Try one week first and see how you feel. You may feel worse before better as gluten is addicting in the brain and your body will experience withdrawal symptoms at first if 100% taken away. One can wean themselves off it as I have successfully.

Cross reactive foods are COFFEE and MILK (DAIRY) products.

Anything refined usually has GLUTEN IN IT,
some examples are:

-cookies
-cereals
-granola
-breads/sandwiches
-bagels
-soups
-dressings
-pizza
-breaded meats
-meat pies
-cakes/pies- desserts
-pastas, noodles
-etc (mostly anything packaged now)

To best avoid the above, try to incorporate **WHOLE (unprocessed)** foods into your diet such as fruits and vegetables, use dips (like yogurt, tahini and lemon, garlic) with vegs., that don't contain gluten, will help make vegs go down. (taste better).
Eat eggs and bacon or fruit and yogurt for breakfast. Have fruit or veg for lunch and soup/salad for dinner. There are several gluten free products out there nowadays due to increased demand and knowledge (tons!!)-6 Billion dollar industry; some at best are only mediocre products so be choosey and read labels!

You can have rice, potatoes, corn (mostly GMO'd), lentils, beans to get carb's and eat a bit of protein. Most experts suggest 1/3 protein in diet.

Snack on nuts, raisins and gogi berries(great for the memory).

"70% of the IMMUNE SYSTEM is in THE GUT !! "

(How gluten affects the body-research says & is very basic here)

You eat gluten, it causes a reaction with the stomach and intestines and body thinks it is an enemy, so attacks it and as it finds it's way into tissues of the body, it causes inflammation as the body begins attacking it. (as I cover inflammation) Eventually your organs and tissues will get damaged, this leads to much pain in the body and fatigue and ailments of all kinds.
I think it affects greatly the mitochondria of cells (energy) (where Mg helps).
It is exhausting when the body is always/constantly fighting something, feels like a constant flu or cold, so thus one feels exhausted and wants to sleep. No energy. Gluten literally destroys the intestines where all the absorption of nutrients from food and supplements takes place. SO even if you are taking the right supplements for your ailment(s), the body will not get them properly with a ruined intestinal system (the micro villi responsible for absorption are flat and destroyed-not working)
So out it goes, money down the toilet, literally.

If you remove the culprit (gluten), the body can slowly begin to heal and instantly you will feel energy as the body is no longer fighting inside and expending energy (mounting an attack against foreign bodies in your body) Eventually the gluten in the tissues is broken down and gotten rid of and pain then dissipates, hormones level out and organs can heal. (the body is really amazing in it's healing abilities and how it can repair damage and regenerate!!)

A friend of mine told me that the reason for so much heart disease is gluten- it causes the arteries to become inflamed and this causes the plaques (clogging of the arteries) whereby once the artery is damaged due to inflammation, plaque builds and builds (to heal inflammation) and this combined with high blood pressure (say due to stress) can cause a heart attack, chest pain or stroke. The pressure(force) of the blood passing a plaque can cause it to peel, break off and be a chunk (clot) that can get stuck anywhere down the line as it travels around, to head, body or heart.

If arteries are kept clean and healthy, plaque does not gather at inflamed sites. Therefore, good blood flow and no big blockages. Yes LDL can help cause clogged arteries but my friend says it begins with the inflammation (which doctors either don't realize or know about), I believe him.

Cholesterol occurs in our bodies in natural amounts (both HDL- good and LDL -"lousy") and people (mainly doctors) make such a big issue of it being the main enemy. It is not. You see when you get the inflammation, the cholesterol will then go there and stick and try to repair the damage, this is where the plaque can form. If one has too much inflammation in arteries (damage) and thusly combined with too much cholesterol then alot of plaques are able to form, this can lead to quadruple bypasses!! etc. To lower ones cholesterol naturally, all one has to do is eat fibre, an apple a day, as the fibre in apples becomes gel like and gathers up cholesterol (cholesterol is attracted to it) and carries it out of the body. This way it can not gather too much and less is available to cause plaques. The real problem is the inflammation caused in the first place by gluten or otherwise. The body is only acting natural in trying to repair it with what it has.

A true fact is that we are not all built the same and some are stronger than others and react differently thus not ALL people react to gluten, just a large segment of the population in which it is growing slowly more and more due to too much long term exposure to this "new" gluten.
When people get too much of something they will naturally build up a sensitivity or allergy to it (right?).

INFLAMMATION

Inflammation can be quite complicated to explain and there are alot of resources out there to explain it in detail, one being wikipedia for instance. However for simplicity sake I will just cover it briefly, what it is, it's purpose and how it impacts fibromyalgia patients.

Inflammation is the process by which we suffer an invader or injury to our body and our body responds sending in troops to try to protect the area. This action results in swelling, redness (extra blood flow to area) and pain as the main ones. Inflammation can result if you cut yourself or break a bone. It also occurs if there are foreign invaders such as an infection the body needs to fend off. The body will react in a cascade of reactions to send the troops to repair and help rid the body of injury or infections.
It is with chronic invaders that chronic inflammation can occur and just as you break a wrist or have a cut, it hurts as the cascade of events happens and **'COX 2' (factor in cascade)** comes into play and causes the pain. Thus you feel pain, so can you with progressive, light inflammation over time. I believe that being allergic or sensitive to food or anything we ingest can be perceived as an invader and this same cascade of events occurs and will induce pain. One such culprit is gluten, if you are gluten sensitive, which alot of people are nowadays due to it's drastic change in structure so that our bodies do not recognize it, the body will attack it and at the same time attack it's own tissues that it inhabits. This is responsible for alot of aches and pain I believe in Fibro people. For others it may be different reasons and just over-excited nerve tissue. I am not too sure. I don't think anyone knows. They say now it all exists in the brain(?)

One thing that truly combats this inflammation pain is Mg as it **inhibits the pain receptors**. This is why I feel when I took alot of Mg when I was in grave pain, the Mg went out into my body and started inhibiting all these receptors so like putting out a fire, the

ambers died down and I could feel better. Makes good sense. I still felt a bit achey and tired until I almost completely got rid of gluten in my diet, then the invader to which I was sensitive and responding to no longer instigated the pain and fatigue. It can be tiring to fight invaders, similar to if you have a bad flu which is what alot of fibro patients will liken their situation to (how they feel).
So in all, if you rid yourself of foreign invaders which in my case seemed to be gluten and when you start to get stronger, other allergens or sensitivities will dissipate and you will not have the bloating (swelling), the redness (skin irritation) and pain in joints and muscles.

Your body will essentially get stronger and more resistant to things it used to react to- less stress on the body and the "fires" in the joints and muscles will go away. You will get proper blood flow, oxygen and the nutrients you feed your body (or it makes) to work optimally. It feels as tho the flu went away, such a good feeling! Over time you will notice a gain in strength and your body change. You may even be back to your old self, or in this case your new self!

GLUTEN AND INFLAMMATION:

Allergy or sensitivity to Gluten can cause inflammation in the body- aches and pains as it attacks the joint tissue.
Inflammation occurs as the body is rejecting something foreign (gluten) and attacks it- this causes inflammation, soon the body is attacking itself as gluten gets stored in tissues.
Gluten is ingested and resides in tissues then the body lodges attacks to rid of it.
Gluten has changed this past 30 years as GMO has modified it to be more refined and cheaper to produce, this has changed it's structure such that people's bodies see it as foreign and an invader, so it attacks it. I have discussed some symptoms of gluten sensitivity previously here.

ARTERIES AND INFLAMMATION:

It is not cholesterol apparently that is the culprit to Heart Disease but rather inflammation of the arteries; when there is an injured artery, such as in inflammation, cholesterol goes in to patch up and recover it, causing plaque buildup (like a scab). Thus it is the injury to the artery that is initial- cholesterol is in the body and collects at sites in the arteries to repair. Statins are big sellers for drug companies so they don't want to disclose the real cause of CAD, big money.

Statins can cause muscle weakness and pain. You need to take COQ10 when taking Statins, as Statins interrupt the ATP cycle and COQ10 helps in this respect.

- 30% of people are intolerant now to gluten
- 5% maybe know or do something about it.

Scientists and researchers have modified and changed our food with technology so it is not the same as in the early 1900's. Our bodies do not recognize it as natural anymore. This leads to illness, CAD, Fibromyalgia, diabetes and maybe even some cancers. Our soil has also changed, with more toxins- overuse of pesticides, hormones and antibiotics.

Gluten is used as fillers now- cheap (all about $). Coffee may mimic gluten in the body- I like non GMO'd coffee, like the brand '365' by Whole Foods.

Cut out pasta, oats and coffee; wheat, barley, oats (cross contamination) and bread.

You may feel worse before you feel better, but inflammation will disappear.

MY STORY WITH GLUTEN:

I have had 10-20 years of fatigue, body aches (all the pressure points), depression (sometimes low level), brain fog, etc. I felt like I was literally dying. Which with a unresolved heart problem I actually was, my systems were weakened by all this. The heart problem was then discovered in my late 20's (29) and fixed , making me feel alot healthier and stronger. Even after being "fixed", I felt fatigue and aches and pains, etc, for years afterwards and this last decade or so. Recently, while working as a Cardiac Tech, I had a patient whereby we discussed gluten inApril 2012. He talked about how much better he felt after removing it, and I agreed I too was sensitive but not ready to make the change. It took me til September 2012 to get it out of my diet, but not completely. I tried one day 100% gluten free from morning til night and the difference I felt was astounding and dramatic- I felt great and healthy, it felt like a miracle occurred. Needless to say I was then sold and started ridding my fridge and diet of the gluten.

In about November 2012 (3 months gluten free) , another patient mentioned to me the book "Wheat Belly". I took an interest as I wished to learn more since I was feeling so much better. Then my mom in the same day mentioned the same book. I immediately, paying attention, went out and purchased it and started reading it as I found I could read books once again and retain information. I was astounded with what I had read. Wheat belly is a book by William Davis, a Cardiologist in Milwaukee. Best book I ever read I thought and was anxious to share his research with all who would listen. It was just 6 months later in January 2013 that I felt completely cured of this dreadful Fibromyalgia.

Six months later (post weaning gluten) all my symptoms disappeared, no more fatigue, I had energy (lots), no more aches and pains in the muscles or joints and brain fog disappeared with it as well as the depression subsiding quite a bit. My mood was also alot better, I was less irritable because no more sugar surges and lows, the fluctuating which often swings peoples moods. (carb's = gluten = sugar)

Now, Jan 2013 I am finishing reading Wheat Belly which talks about wheat and it's detrimental effects on health. You will find all you need to know in great detail by reading the book but right here I will cover some basics.

Basically wheat has changed (GMO- genetically modified organism) from it's nearly pure, simple and natural form to something not digested nor utilized by the human body and leads to inflammation and all kinds of diseases, especially modern day ones on the rise, namely diabetes being the biggest one. (and gluten seems to be in everything!) William Davis touches on gluten being responsible for things like fibromyalgia which reinforced my theory even more. It seemed like a very plausible culprit indeed. It is thru my experience I became convinced. As one is unsure til they live thru something and thusly know the difference. Not all people are affected in the same way, so for some this may make no sense and for others complete and logical sense, we are all individuals.

When one gets inflammation in the body it causes in turn extreme pain and fatigue thus it is seen as an enemy entering the body and the body is under attack similar to a flu bug and eventually will attack itself (the body and systems). **It causes the nerves to be overactive and oversensitive, thus the pain to touch.**

WHEAT AND THE BRAIN :

Wheat is very addicting to the brain and an appetite stimulant (you just want more of it). It is similar to being on drugs as you become dopey and foggy, the brain is under attack as the gluten, in it's simple form, crosses the Brain Blood Barrier and attaches itself to opiate receptors, giving one a high, a feeling of euphoria and satisfaction. This also leads to depression which Wheat Belly I believe covers well. Mg has been proven to help with depression.

The wheat (gluten) when it breaks down causes sugar surges and then a huge low, like a roller coaster, unlike protein which is slowly broken down and keeps the blood sugar steady. This up and down is very bad for diabetics and pre-diabetics alike. It also is broken down so quickly that there is too much for the body to turn into energy that it then stores it as visceral fat in the belly and around organs. When we gain this fat we gain weight and size. It is stored energy, similar to filling your car with a full tank of gas when it only uses a little at a time. Wheat makes us "feel" fat and bloated as well. I think as it is so toxic it helps retain water in the tissues (bloating). Even when I eat a little and cheat I afterwards feel very bloated and I even see the belly on myself, all my wt. loss gone to pieces. So beware of having even a little and cheating, it will surely make you feel bloated and irritable.

Having a tummy like this up front is bad for the body. Tummy fat is bad for diabetics whereas, I once read, the buttocks fat and coffee (to some degree) help prevent diabetes.

GLUTEN AND THE TUMMY:

Gluten causes bloating and a tummy like you are pregnant. This fat that accumulates is bad for diabetes and it causes all the hormones to go out of balance so one does not feel good and this fat is so negative for the body. Personally I encountered thyroid problems (hypothyroidism) when I found myself eating more gluten, I think gluten helped destroy it's function and the thyroid (in the neck) is **vital** to hormone balance in the body. Getting rid of gluten and exercise can rid you of the tummy and diabetes will then not become an issue and hormones will be less interrupted in the body. I think the hormone Estrogen is greatly affected – the belly fat makes more, can lead to mood swings, depression and irritability. Apparently this fat gives off what are called Estrones. (stores them).

Eat Kale, brocolli and cabbage to help combat it. I have covered Estrogen and it's relationship to Fibromyaglia earlier.

Wheat nowadays in it's unnatural and over- GMO'd form causes many modern day diseases from chronic heart disease , to cancer, to immune disease (70% of the immune system is in the gut, which gluten destroys the gut!), to diabetes, all on the rise. Drug co.'s are making alot of money from this, be sure!

We treat disease nowadays , due to modern western medicine and their belief in black and white thinking, that we treat the disease with a PILL to make it lessen vs. finding out the underlying cause and creating health instead of managing disease. Disease is not an enemy, it is actually your friend, it is trying to teach us something. Just as our body rejects wheat in it's new form, it is telling us it is no good. One must not "fight" disease but rather "create" health. Get to know your disease like you would a friend so that you may help it.

By getting rid of wheat one can start creating health and thus the body will repair itself as it has astounding and god-like abilities(especially to recover itself). Just get to the root cause.

You must be your own doctor and educate yourself, become an expert on your illness. A good doctor will listen to you as a team, if he/she doesn't, find one that will. You, after all, know yourself best.

So how do you know if you are gluten sensitive or gluten intolerant, easy take this test.

1. do you have a belly that won't go away?
2. are you irritable?
3. do you drink alot of coffee to stimulate yourself?
4. are you tired all the time?
5. are you achey?
6. do you have brain fog?
7. do you suffer depression?
8. are you addicted to carb's, esp gluten?

General stuff I know, but this is how gluten presents itself, in a general way. Then your body, when it cannot take it anymore, reacts with a specific disease, whether heart attack (due to atherosclerosis) or diabetes or cancer. It crosses the line from general to specific as it attacks systems in the body one at a time, whichever is weakest (genetically or otherwise).

A real test to see if you are gluten sensitive/intolerant is just go off of it for 3 weeks to 6 weeks and see if you feel even a bit better, reaching for less coffee, less irritable, no more bloated feeling.
It may be gradual on some, it is all individual depending how sensitive you are or how much damage exists in the body. Try it, what do you have to lose, your belly??

So what I encourage for Fibromyalgia is to take Mg to settle the overactive nerves and cramps and cut out gluten either by weaning off of or cold turkey (cold turkey best for most). I weaned myself, allowing gradual disappearance of gluten to where I am 90 % gluten free now (no one is perfect!). What I did to replace gluten for texture and carb intake was make gluten free pancakes for breakfast for a couple months and do also a bit of rice (brown or white) pasta the odd dinner. Then I did not feel like

I missed it so much. Soon my body was recovering without me suffering from gluten loss. I now do no more gluten -free pancakes (only as a treat) and have lowered my carb intake as it still has a high glycemic index and can cause surges of blood sugar and some fat to accumulate.

A slow process for sure but soon you will notice it easier to find gluten free food and that your addiction to gluten lessens or disappears. You will eventually come to hate gluten and see it as a poison, an enemy to the body and will not enjoy having it at all. I still have gluten days, maybe one-day or meal every 3 weeks but I hope to do none one day. Certainly it is tempting and very difficult to avoid in today's world especially when one is looking to spend less on groceries. But remember , your health is an investment, protect it!

It is primarily because North America took on feeding 3rd world countries with grain and had to produce alot of it and for cheap that we have apparently found ourselves with this high-yielding , disease resisting wheat.

I believe at minimum our food should be labelled as GMO as to give each consumer the knowing of what they are ingesting- only fair, let the consumer decide, not the manufacturer. In Europe, I believe, they must all be labelled. We should push for it and follow suit, our healthcare crisis and the business of it all is out of control and in the long run costs us much more $$ and pain, suffering and loss.

As well, I believe people (drug co's) should not be allowed to patent something nature made and is an organism, whether plant or animal (ie. Gluten/wheat).

Some people say only 10% of the population are gluten sensitive. I think it is more like 30-40% of the pop. (this is more realistic, as you being aware after reading wheat belly, you look around and see how many do really suffer- it is high).

When I have gluten now I will feel flu like symptoms, tired and achey but just for a bit til my body rids it. I will also crave more gluten in the same day.

I hope this approach helps you as it did me, it is in no way meant as medical advice nor to replace medical advice.

Just an experienced and educated opinion.

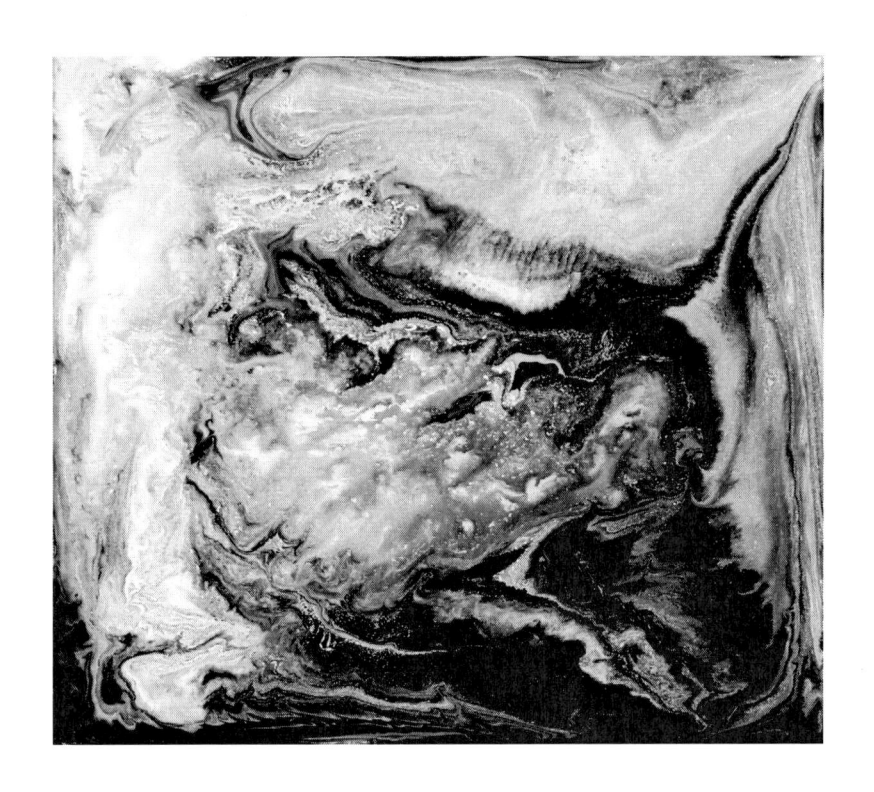

PART 2- FIBRO MANAGED

VIII. Fibro Symptoms & Vitamins that work.
Depression, Stress, Mood, Fatigue and Pain

DEPRESSION:

Depression is a part of fibro whether it comes first or later. Some people with fibro take a small amount of antidepressants. Depression is a very difficult illness as there are no real tests for it to show, say your significant other, just a deep dark hole of hopelessness one feels. No one can physically see it so they always tell you-just pull yourself up by your bootstraps, at least my mom says this. It is not the mere blues but a possible chemical imbalance in the brain and thus the whole body. Brain chemicals are out of sync and this also throws off a persons hormones I believe, making one irritable as well. (The brain and Hormones are intimately intertwined). One can feel tired and blue in the brain and then in the body, you can develop aches and pains and great fatigue. You lack the motivation to even shower at times. Self neglect may set in. No one seems to understand yet so many of us experience this- like we are alone in the dark. No one discusses it- how we really feel.

WHY DEPRESSION SO PREVALENT AND ON THE RISE TODAY: (#1 is stress)

Our society is evermore so segregated and isolated then ever before. People have their own jobs, cliques and families which they stick to and while it creates independence, it isolates one like in a cocoon , not needing others to get by. Social interaction is a very important factor for humans and especially feeling connected to a community. Commonly, while the rich get richer they isolate themselves even more as paranoia about others misusing them grows; this can lead to the sadness many rich people experience.

Besides isolation, our society is so fear based now and consumer based. We are more interested in how much stuff or how many houses we can accumulate instead of how many friends. Chasing the almighty dollar which we think will make us happy. True happiness exists in the simple act of sharing whether it be time, patience, skills, comfort, conversation, help or guidance (sharing money too!). Not in stuff. Stuff is just alot of work and alot of the time "empty". Sure when we first get it, we enjoy it because it is "new" and "foreign" but then we grow bored and forget we have or own it. The high is gone too quick.

So this lack of dependence on each other and accumulation of stuff leads to ultimately empty feelings and loneliness and alot of stress, internal and external. Most people don't have hobbies anymore, something to relieve stress. I relieve stress with doing art, my creativity, some read, some watch tv (entertainment). Also with the evolution of social media we are more plugged in than ever and stressed out. We have no time for play- people need to just unplug and regain grounding and sense.

Number two of why depression is on the rise may be the stigma people experience when we discuss mental illness. I know no one with a 100% healthy mind, minus Dr. Oz perhaps. If we don't speak and share knowledge and experience then things don't get resolved, they get worse.
 So we judge, with mental illness we perceive people who have it to be weak and possibly sinners (some religions). Most who do battle it are some of the strongest people I've ever met. As when you don't have your mind, you have nothing. That is hard. Even a person in a wheelchair with a healthy mind is far better off than a person with a "functioning body but sick mind". The mind guides us. It has to be healthy . We think a thought then feel an emotion and if our thoughts are not healthy, neither are our emotions. And if our emotions are not healthy then neither are our bodies, they become toxic and sick too. Then nothing functions. That is why it is so important to think positively, to dream, to hope, to be optimistic, no matter what the challenge. And always think the best of things and people, it will make for a happier and healthier you, even if you end up being a little off base.

People need to talk about depression like they do cancer and now aids-openly and honestly. We may soon find we are not alone and this in itself gives us much needed comfort and support. People who overcome mental challenges and obstacles should be celebrated as there are so few quick fixes and solutions, often the journey is long and solutions largely unknown. So much to still learn about the brain and research still has a long way to go. If we put as much resources into mental health as we do things like cancer there would be more hope for many people and this could lead to better health and societal contribution.

I believe communication between humans is vital to healthy relationships and education (learning). We are not mind readers nor can any one of us have ALL the answers. We must share what we know and help find answers.

DEPRESSION:

SHOULD YOU BE ON ANTI-DEPRESSANTS ?......

I talk quite a bit here about anti- depressants and read with caution as you should always consult with a doctor, but I guarantee you that almost 90-100% of Fibromyalgia patients are on an anti-depressant. (even low level).
If you have "mild" depression it is a popular belief now that you not be on any sort of anti-depressants and that this can make things worse for you. You have to weigh out the benefits vs. the risks of taking something, especially when it has such a powerful effect on the brain and harsh side effects. Talk with your doctor or preferably a psychiatrist when it comes to fiddling with your brain. Depression can sometimes just simply be a symptom and not a cause and in the case of fibro it is a symptom. So what I suggest one do is other things to battle the depression, such as

EXERCISE
EPA- OMEGA FATS (fish oil)
PSYCHOTHERAPY- talk therapy
TAKE Mg
VITAMIN D
take Curcumin- in tumeric

This will help with little, if any, side effects.

Some facts about anti-depressants are:

— since 1987 when Prozac was first introduced, today it is a multi-billion dollar business and **at least** 1 out of 10 of us are on one- that is approx. 30 million Americans.

— With a total of 40 million Americans (minimum) using antidepressants, 1.7 Billion annually is spent on that alone where psychiatry is an 8 billion dollar industry annually.

Antidepressants:
- can cause nauseau, sexual dysfunction and suicide.
- may change the brain.
- family doctors are actually encouraged to prescribe antidepressants.
- FDA warns for children and adolescents, there is a suicide warning. Can make one manic too which can lead to problems.
- one out of 4 women between age of 40-60 are on one. A 400% increase over the past several years.
- May get depression back and worse.
- No evidence depression is related to low serotonin levels.
- Anti-depressants causes chemical imbalances in the brain leading at times to increased confusion, impulsiveness and irritability.
— Brain trauma can cause depression.
- 75% of usage is "off label use", meaning is issued for:
    -insomnia,
    -migraines or
    -weight loss,
where there is no evidence it helps with any of these. The first two solved with Mg actually. Maybe even wt. loss too, as Mg gives energy.

FIBROSUCCESS

One can have depression as a **_SYMPTOM_** (not cause) of:
- Anaemia
- PCOS (poly cystic ovarian syndrome)
- PMS
- Low thyroid
- Celiac disease
- Fibro and pain

For drug companies to get a drug approved for use and sale, they only need 2 clinical trials showing _slight_ improvement over use of a placebo, they could have 20 trials that say otherwise or are harmful but these are not introduced to Health Canada or the FDA. They only show the positive results, not negative, seems a little deceptive if you ask me.

- Also Health Canada division for drug approval is run (paid for) by drug companies as they pay for it, so of course "we" will let them do what they wish. Antidepressants have only a 10% rate of efficacy in the general population meaning that it works for that segment, the other 90% of the population, it is virtually useless and a possible hazard (especially now they are finding for adolescents). So think twice before you get sold on taking an antidepressant, try magnesium first instead if it is mild and your doctor says is ok, tell your doctor about other methods to help your depression that you have learned about. Work together. Exercise is super beneficial, if you can.

People are on antidepressants and shouldn't be, even when you get off, you will carry a "label"(stigma) around from doctor to doctor and with insurance companies the rest of your life, so think wisely before you are prescribed one and make sure other important workups are performed beforehand. If you need to wean yourself off of them, do so with the help of a doctor as it is no fun and very hard with withdrawal symptoms, similar to getting off coffee but worse. Whatever you do do not go cold turkey, could lead to seizures in the brain!

So in conclusion if you are on an antidepressants, and really don't need it, they can cause all sorts of problems with your brain activity and functioning, throwing off normal chemicals. Make sure then that depression is the cause for you and not just a symptom of something else. If you are suicidal or have deep depression, then the antidepressants are recommended as they do help save lives if depression is the primary cause. Please talk to your doctor about.

Note: This is in no way meant to replace medical advice.

MEDICATIONS VS. NATURAL REMEDIES FOR DEPRESSION:

Medications have a long way to go however, there are good natural remedies that help depression a great deal. I am not discounting drugs though because when you finally find one that works for you, it feels like a cure (but have side effects). With natural remedies there seem to be less extreme side effects, if any. Probably one of the most unrealized natural remedies to help is **Fish Oil-Omega 3's**-your brain needs these like the body needs water. It nourishes the brain, like oil for a car- it can't run without it.

In brief: (what scientifically helps)

FISH OIL- imagine your brain as a big gel mass, it needs oil as part of it's contents- it keeps it running- I use Nordic fish oil or Nutrasea- liquid, usually one teaspoon/day, anytime usually in the AM.

EXERCISE - scientifically helps. It is proven that exercise helps release serotonin in the brain, the feel good chemical. It also helps your body find and flush out toxins by getting the blood flowing.
So helps cleanse the body. Circulation is improved.

VITAMIN D- scientifically helps. It has been shown that Vitamin D deficiency in the brain can lead to psychosis. It is called the "Sunshine Vitamin" and we all need that. Thus it assists with SADS- seasonal affective disorder. Take about 2000 IU /day (or ask a nutritionist). Need Mg to absorb Vitamin D.

B VITAMINS- these are to combat stress. I myself for years have taken B12 shots once- twice /month and I take a B multivitamin. B's help the brain keep calm. (B6 is important for women.)

EVENING PRIMROSE OIL (EPO)- Helps with mood- PMS in particular so if you are irritable, a very good one to take , calms the body and mind right down- you become less toxic and angry for sure. A miracle for mood. (mainly for if high estrogen levels) If you have a tummy, you likely need EPO. Ultra Prim-Omega Factors brand is the one I use.

* **Curcumin**: an important spice found in Turmeric, it is now concluded thru studies that 500 Mg taken twice daily can help you as much as an antidepressant does. You can buy in capsule form.

SLEEP- we all need rest, I get 6-8 hours minimum. Sleep is when the body repairs and rejuvenates itself. It stops or slows all functions.
The odd nap never hurt anyone and recharges the brain.

WATER- dehydration can lead to hallucinations and delusions. The brain and body needs hydration. If you are sensitive to tap water, drink a good mineral water or try filtering and putting it in the fridge to cool. I drink a minimum 1 litre/day. Most people recommend 8 glasses/day. Hydrating helps when you feel blue. When you put H2O in the fridge for about 20 min, chlorine is a volatile gas and will dissipate so you will not be able to taste it.

PET-good companion- unconditional love. Loving an animal opens the soul and fills our mind with flowing positive thoughts and feelings- is very healing.

TRACE MINERALS- I am not sure what purpose this serves exactly, however, these trace minerals found in sea salt , etc are REQUIRED for cells to function even at all. We only need tiny amounts. I use Himilayan sea salt when I cook.

ZINC- I take this for my brain. It is required I believe in alot of energy transfers. Recently I learned that if you up your zinc your testosterone levels increase and this decreases cortisol levels & lowers stress. But be careful with too much Zinc as you may fall victim to copper deficiency as it interrupts absorption of. I also learned that Zinc helps keep your hair from graying.

JOURNAL- I use this to release toxic thoughts and getting it out in a harmless way is healthy. (won't destroy relationships).

CARBS - It has been stated that **carbs help increase serotonin** in the brain and help get a good nights sleep. If you do no carbs, I would add a bit to your diet. I know I watch my intake carefully due to wt. Gain. Carbs can have a high glycemic index.

You can use naturally whatever you find to work , the above is just suggestions and core basics, some proven by science to help work for depression. It can help one alleviate their depression, it helps the body heal itself by doing daily activities and even exercise and getting out and socializing. Living Life.

Diverting your attention when you are depressed:

I have found in the past that it helps to divert your brain off of the topic that is making you feel depressed and sad which keeps circulating in your brain, like you can't get out. First of all if something has disturbed you or broken you , find a solution to it and make a plan, feel positive and optimistic that things will get better or resolved. Be optimistic again. Even write down this plan if you have to, the solving of the situation will divert your brain off of the problem. You will go from a problem to a solution. Try also to minimize the problem in your mind, making the mountain into a mole hill. Once you formulate a solution then indulge in a happy hobby or just go out with a friend to get your mind off of things. This will in fact give your mind a rest and make you feel a lot happier and relaxed. Then have a good sleep and give your brain more rest, thinking happy thoughts before you drift off asleep, even journal if you need to.

In the morning post breakdown you should be feeling a lot better, optimistic and back to your old self again with the problem not so overwhelming and looming in your brain.
Spend the next few days doing activities you enjoy, taking a break from real life if you can. Have in your head the idea that you will implement the plan after a few days to not feel you are in such a hurry and add stress to the situation, just tuck the 'plan' away for a bit. Within these next few days you should snap out of it, at minimum have a grip on the situation and feel more relaxed and in control of your brain. Thus depression and the state of being in it will not be the central issue in your life or thinking, it will not have that powerful grasp it tends to have.

While the above may not be enough I am supportive of some antidepressants as I believe in a mix of western and eastern medicine-both in balance are beneficial. Your doctor can help you decide the best one for you. You may only need for a period of time til your brain regains it's health and can function on it's own.

I firmly believe the brain or any organ in your body can heal or recover from injury or illness. Your brain will definately function better when your gut functions better too!
(70% serotonin is produced in the gut!)

STRESS – "STRESS IS CONTAGIOUS!!"

Stress, there is helpful stress (positive) and unhealthy stress (negative); when it motivates you, that is healthy, when it overwhelms and hurts you, that is unhealthy. People with fibro are often worse with added stress, it may go from a 5 to a 9 or 10 on the pain scale when you add stress. Stress creates havoc with the body, it creates adrenalin which helps the body move and think to a degree but when you slip over the line of too much adrenalin it damages the body and systems to a great degree, including the brain.

With Fibro, stress heightens pain, sensitivities and depression. We feel alot more fatigue and pain. Anything can stress us- family, work, finances, relationships that are toxic or negative, friends,children, having too much stuff, no hobby to turn to, etc. Everyone has different stressors and reacts differently too- you just have to know your body and what triggers the discomfort. Stress can be internal or external. Stress can come from just sitting in a room alone thinking negatively. You think the worst will happen so this result may stress you. This is why meditation and positive thinking is so important. As when you have a fearful thought in your brain, your body reacts with emotion and this triggers chemicals to race thru your body-whether adrenalin or endorphins- we go into fight or flight mode. You must learn to calm your mind and understand how you perceive yourself, your environment and surroundings. Meditation and yoga are very helpful at this as it forces you to calm, stop and redirect. It is very grounding.

Stress, I believe, literally destroys the body and is likely the cause of all illnesses including to a great degree cancer. When we are weak or weakened, that is when the bad things in our bodies can take over whether it be cancer cells, bacteria, virus, blood sugars, etc. Anything your body can normally keep at bay and in control goes out of whack. We must strive to keep our bodies as strong and fit as they can genetically be. We must understand our bodies weaknesses and practice to strengthen them. Your body is a tool you must keep in top performing order, just like a machine or car for instance if you wish it to work best. I believe we have soul/spirits and our bodies are our tool whereby our souls are able to carry out their purpose, whatever that may be, whether it be the brain (mental) or physical (body) functioning at optimum levels whereby we assist others who are not so fortunate or have other skills.

NURTURING OUR OWN BODIES

So therefore we must nurture and care for and honour our tool (body) with all we know. We are all here for a reason and purpose and eventually most figure that out, some often too late in life as we are conditioned to perform like robots at suboptimal levels. So if one can decrease stress or get it to a healthy level where it just motivates you then your body can begin to heal and get stronger and serve you better and illness will eventually disappear. There is this one story of this woman who was diagnosed with stage 4 terminal cancer whereby medicine would only make it worse, they took a wait and see approach, after some time she spontaneously healed and was in complete remission, she stated she just began putting herself first and letting go of all the stress. She must of centred herself and began feeling positive and relaxing with things. This is amazing what one can achieve when they realize what is not working and take the steps to fix it.
She did not at first realize by changing her priorities and thinking, that this would help heal the cancer but I believe it did. The doctors are still unsure how this happened but I am not - The mind

is super powerful and releasing stress can do wonders to assist the body in it's daily battles.

We must all take responsibility and must mostly become your own doctor and trust your own instincts by educating yourself on how you feel and what is known to help and then by trial and error. It all takes time and patience. If you need "time out" from the cycle of life to do this too - then take it- take a sabbatical if you can or do it as daily practice while you work more healthy.

Not everyone has the opportunity I have such as time, in that way I am very rich, as I have the time to pay attention, shut out all negativity and heal. I normally work 2 days/ wk with 5 days off. Often when one gets something like Fibro, it is so serious that one becomes disabled and must go on disability and take time off to heal or just be. Use this time to your advantage if you are given it or even the little bits you can find in life-indulge yourself, take a class, take a nap, dance, play, meditate, read, do a hobby, some time out for yourself so you may de-stress. Even thinking about going on a holiday, somewhere nice and warm is relaxing and invigorating. Even if just a dream, the thought is positive and calming. At least if you have no time in your life to do all this , take Mg and de-Calcify your body, and try stopping gluten, the pain will go away and it will help calm your mind.

SOME COMMON STRESS FACTORS :

- work too much or too little.
-caffeine (stimulants)
-negative thinking
-being unhappy
-toxic family or friends or bosses
-too busy: overwhelmed
-type A personality
-perfectionist

-lack of sleep (deep sleep)
-no release
-no hobby
-no "me-time"
-diet-lack of vitamins/minerals
-too much "stuff" to look after
-FINANCES (debt)
-lack of social, friends, community
-traffic (commute); computers (plugged in)
-being unhappy, trapped, stuck
-raising children, looking after aging parents
-lack of planning, goals
-ILLNESS, esp. long term

You have to carefully see each of the above as triggers and try to resolve what you can or at least control them. There may be different ones for each person but these are the main ones I feel we deal with in our day and age. Feel free to discover your own.

Vitamins and stuff for stress:

Ashwaganda- for adrenals/stress/cortisol
Evening Primrose Oil- for mood
Mg + - calming on muscles and brain, takes away aches/pains
Holy basil and Rhodoila- adrenals, stress.
Less coffee - less adrenalin (fight or flight), for nerves.
Lemon Balm- acts like valium, calms the mind
B Vitamins- combats stress
Vitamin C- neutralizes cortisol
L-Theanine- calms down the mind

MENTAL STRESS:

A big source of mental stress is when we make things in our mind bigger than they actually are-mountains out of molehills. A friend of mine actually was driving herself crazy because she made a tiny, negligible mistake at work one day which she assumed would get her fired. So she lost sleep, had panic attacks, drove herself nutso. After one week of intense stress, after she told her boss, it turned out her boss really did not even care. I myself, turned this international exam I had into such a big deal, I put it off for 8-9 months so I could study enough, when it came down to it, I studied one week periodically, went in calmly thinking "ok this is just practice, I can rewrite it"- well I aced it with 93%. It was actually so easy. I built it up into something it wasn't, it became so overwhelming.
So silly how I put it off, stressed and wasted precious time. We all do this type of thing to ourselves.

It is often better too , when things are big, downplay them in your mind and as well keep the small things, small. Our minds can run out of control if we let it, and this releases chemicals into our bodies which are destructive. It is all about perception and interpreting realistically. (Even if we have to lie to ourselves, in the end we usually have little control over outcomes anyhow, so why stress?)

STRESS AND HYDRATION:
Stress can lead to dehydration as when your nervous you get thirsty, I don't know the exact mechanism of why this happens but know it does. When we stress the enzymes in our mouths (and guts) decrease so this could be the reason, and this can lead to more cavities as the moist enzymes help keep bacteria at bay. This may be why you see people who are constantly stressed with bad teeth.
When we dehydrate and feel thirsty, our brains can suffer, can cause cloudy thinking and/or lead to mental breakdowns. The

brain needs fluids. So stay heavily hydrated especially during times of stress whether high or ongoing. Water and good water (mineral H2O) is the best and most important thing you put in your body. Our bodies and especially our brains cannot function properly without it.

THERE ARE "3" UNADVOIDABLE ASPECTS OF HUMAN NATURE WHICH HELP <u>INDUCE STRESS</u>:

1. we all want what we Don't have.
2. we React
3. we all need a sense of Control.

1. WE ALL WANT WHAT WE DON'T HAVE.

This attitude stresses us out as we strive to get what others seem to have and at the same time are not thankful for what we already do have. If we just relax and be happy and very thankful for the blessings that surround us (what we already have) then life flows alot easier and we focus on positivity, happiness and joy. Being thankful is very healthy, it gives us a feeling of fulfilment and contentment. This in itself reduces stress as we stop working so hard for those things that others might possess, which may not even be possible for us too.

One small example is a friend I have who has beautiful spirally curly blond hair, she wishes it was straight and me, I wish I had her hair, but in the end I think to myself, look I am happy I just have hair, straight or curly, it is nice and I am thankful for it.

When we stop chasing unobtainable or difficult desires we **think** will make us happy, we feel alot more relaxed and slowdown in life and smell the roses. The stress seems to go away.

2. WE REACT.

This is big as when we react we have to spend all this energy on putting out the fires we caused by reacting or blowing our fuse. This in itself takes alot of already limited energy. So how do we not react you ask?....you think first before you react, take a breath, god gave us brains to think before we leap into action, no?.....we have this ability vs. animals. When we take a step back and decide that what is going on has to do with the other person and not me and NOT take it personally as an attack, we tend to act differently and more logically. We cannot be angry and thankful at the same time, so always count your blessings. This problem of reacting is in part tied into #3. We all need a sense of control.

3. WE ALL NEED A SENSE OF CONTROL.

Yes whether it is controlling our children's behaviour or their future, we all try to have control. If we just realize we have very little control over the universe minus our own behaviour, action, and future, then things become easier. Giving up this having to "have control" over people, family, friends, kids, jobs, or situations is liberating. We have to still have sense of responsibility but stop trying to control what others say or how they behave in order to have our own sense of power, unless of course someone is acting very disrespectful or bullying another then it is time to step in a bit and not be apathetic.

Again, we have to realize that most what people say and do has to do with themselves personally and not us. I find it very stress free when I think that all I have to control is myself. Yes we can give people sometimes much needed direction but ultimately we have to see that it is in everyone's own hands to do as they will. This act of realizing what we truly have control over will dissipate much unnecessary expended stress.

STRESS AND KISSING:

It has actually been studied that if one kisses alot in life, that they can extend their lifespan by 5 years. Yes kissing is healthy. Firstly when a woman kisses a man there is testosterone in the mans saliva which then enters the women via mouth, this testosterone helps lower cortisol levels as discussed in the adrenal burnout section, thus the women calms down and feels a sense of de-stress. As well the act of kissing releases Oxytocin in a woman and Oxytocin is the same hormone that is released when a woman gives childbirth, thus the deep attachment woman will feel when they kiss another person. Oxytocin is a feel good hormone and again very calming. When one gets their feet massaged the same release of Oxytocin can occur. I believe that kissing a pet has the same impact on the brain in that we can release Oxytocin , thus the connection we feel towards pets that develops, much as if they were a child. It is very healthy then just to kiss your pet, pending you are not allergic!
Kissing a pet can be calming and make you feel good, reducing stress and helping relieve the mind.
Therefore whether you kiss a human or pet, I have this listed under the topic stress and is classified here as a stress reducer.

Emotional Health connected to Physical Health

We all know the mind, body and spirit are connected but nothing is so strong as when we emotionally suffer and it manifests into physical ailments or pain. If one shuts down something painful it becomes insomnia or migraines, or worse ulcers and can build up toxicity in the body even causing what I believe, cancers at worst. My aunt is suffering so emotionally right now as she hates where she lives and has money issues etc, that her kidneys are shutting down, her lungs are congested and she is in alot of pain. She was at a breaking point mentally too. They are tied together as you don't deal with something that bothers you , it builds in your mind, causes physical pain and then this physical pain causes you more mental anguish and concern (worry).

Iyanla Vazant was on Dr. Oz recently and she talked about it being tied together as well and she had good advice: feel, deal and heal. I guess this means acknowledge and allow yourself to feel, let it flow thru and out of your body, deal with what it is causing you it (whether you need to change jobs, have a talk with someone, etc), take steps to eradicate the negative feeling and then Heal, allow yourself the time and space to get better and recover from it's destruction in you spiritually, mentally and physically. Healing thoughts that keep you present. The body can recover, if you allow it. Don't stay stuck because it is familiar to you, nothing worse. She stated we all need to feel acknowledged, seen and valued, especially I feel as women as we do so much for others and little gets acknowledged if any. And women are such emotional creatures vs. Men, we tend to have more emotional/physical afflictions than they do (maybe why also Fibro more evident in women). It is a proven structural thing in the brain that we FEEL more and process more than men. (just generalizing mind you).

Iyanla stated 3 reasons we feel emotional pain and these are also 3 challenges: they are,

1. Fear of not being loved.
2. Fear of not being seen, heard or valued
3. Fear of not having an authentic voice (speak what you want/feel). Be true to yourself is what I gather here.

Feelings are simply energy: If they are toxic you need to release them, welcome them, acknowledge them and breathe thru it, if you need to sweat it out, go and exercise to release all that negativity and it will just flow out, it needs a place to go and like if you pent up explosives and then a match gets lit, it explodes like pent up negative feelings do. Tho most of us will not explode, we will just simply shut down emotionally and get stuck and then this will show eventually in illness and physical pain. Toxicity is not good for anyone. <u>All feelings carry with it energy</u> and this can be positive if you are happy, this is often very productive energy and you feel like sharing it with others or doing something celebratory to release it, but often if it is negative we feel ashamed to share it and thus don't release it and often it can manifest in bad habits such as overeating, overspending, drinking, drug use , etc, all bad for you. So, acknowledging it , giving it respect and releasing it is very important, essentially, and we have all heard this "let- it-go".

Like a bad friend, if they do you nothing but harm you would let them go as a healthy decision , so why not do the same with toxic emotions, they do not serve you in a healthy positive way and sometimes can be contagious as we all sense stress and negativity around us. So just let it go , however you may have to do that, but either meditate, tell a friend you trust with it, journals are always very beneficial here or exercise it out.

What works is "let people support you" and decide if "the fear of doing something different is greater than the maximal pain you feel"(when you are stuck). Try to build a community of support around you.

We all deal with negative and toxic feelings , no one is immune as we are all human and with good comes bad and visa-versa, so learn to not hide or suppress it, it is part of stigma people don't talk about problems they are having but really we are all in this world together and all have individual skills that benefit each other. People need to share more and communicate and respect when someone feels bad, we all don't want to hear about it cause we are afraid it will bring us down, but maybe your offer of advice will help that person release or figure a way out and that will make everyone feel better. I talk about stigma here in this book and how damaging this "judgement of others" really is and can be.

Stigma with depression: "stigma sucks!"

There is just no good in having stigma, it prevents resolution and hope. As humans, it is in our nature to judge and fear (esp fear based in 21 st century-media) but we are also creatures of habits and conditioning, and if we are fed enough negative energy and news about a topic it will induce this stigma and judgement to a nth degree where it becomes difficult to now undo. We are such that most do not trust their instincts because we can't see them and thus we question them. We always make mistakes when we go against our instincts as instincts are really our higher and truer self speaking to us via feelings (energy). If we cannot see it, we don't believe it and when it comes to illness this can be a very painful judgement for those who suffer and it is not visible, we all look for physical cues, like a cane, a wheelchair, a limp, a sad face, a skinny/fat body before we acknowledge there may be a problem and usually at this stage it has become too late.

Stigma hurts those who suffer from Fibro because you cannot see it, so people don't believe you but like a diabetic you cannot see that in a person, at least I cannot tell one by looking at them but when they say they are diabetic, we immediately just believe them, surely they can't be faking it, there are blood tests.

As with Fibro, people question the illness cause there is no definitive test to show you are in pain and suffering. Sure there are those in life, very few numbers, who will fake something but in thinking this is everyone, imagine how much you hurt those who are real sincere, it doesn't serve them well. It makes it more difficult and harder and often become worse with less support or help. Stigma is strongly evident in mental illness, because often if we cannot acknowledge it by a simple test, we disregard it. I just feel science is not good enough yet with the brain to definitely show what we as humans need to physically see. Brain scans are getting much better but there is still no simple blood test.

People with mental illness, (and in Fibro many sufferers, if not all, deal with depression which even low level is hard to deal with), are questioned too often about how they hurt and they have trouble expressing it because

a. No one will listen
b. No one wants to understand
c. No one knows solutions

We understand the heart so very well that they are transplanting no problem now, they are building hearts from scratch and there are so many solutions for anything that ails the heart. People immediately feel sorry for you when it comes to a heart problem and heart attacks and it's so freely discussed, they get nothing but support, help and answers. Why such a difference with the illness of the brain, the brain deserves immense respect as it is boss when it comes to the body, it has almost full control, it is all neurons , our computer hardware. We need to put money into mental health initiatives & get less stigmatized about it. It is the most horrible thing in the world. Actually, the most horrible thing about it is how people treat you when they learn you do not have a perfect, healthy brain- stigma, they run away and judge, no pity, no support.

And to be honest with you no one has a perfect brain, it is not black and white whether you are healthy or ill, alot of grey area and we can all be a little "off". It takes alot of compassion and 'benefit of the doubt behaviour' that a certain behaviour is not on purpose, but rather the brain acting out. With stigma, dialogue solves all I feel and if we can put our shields and judgement down, toss them to the side and just talk and learn, share, help and really support and believe people who suffer mentally, we would go a long ways to a stronger community.
The media plays a tremendous and important role in forming our thoughts, judgements and fears, they always have stories on that are negative about people with mental illness, that they are all

hurtful and evil and do wrong, well the truth is that it is a very small segment and it gets blown outta proportion often.

There are alot of strong, loving, contributing, gentle, giving, smart, soft souls who suffer mental illness but it is never exposed or talked about, cause it is not dramatic enough or they fear the stigma of being outed, so don't speak up. People feed into drama, we all love it as it feels exciting and we like the rush it gives us. I personally like being mellow and avoid drama cause that is all it is, something overblown and dramatized. They should make it illegal to disclose public health situations on the media, they do not say for instance one of the gang members had cancer and that is why he shot another. (that would be odd) Well so is it odd we think all people with mental problems are dangerous and are throw away citizens.

Mental illness can be a gift, it is actually a higher functioning brain and if science could figure out why and how it occurs, they will discover it happens often to very intelligent and sensitive people (higher functioning) whose brains are just going into over active drive at times. (some mental illnesses can be triggered by illegal drugs, that is not what I discuss here) True there can be violent people who are mental but this group is actually very small and mental does not equate to violent which is what people believe. When people "think" you are violent or doing/saying bad things 'on purpose' they will avoid you or try to hurt you in defence , this is not what most mental people need at all.

Support gives people strength whether it just be a hug, a new drug that helps or just talking(to release or sort out). Our brains remain quite mysterious and complicated but if we can figure out computers and create them (which in essence act like brains) surely we can solve the problems of the brain and this lead to healthier, more fulfilled lives.

Mental illness is only rising in numbers too, it is not falling, as we have not helped fix it and people are more and more breaking under the stress of our modern day world and bad diet. Nutrition is key and as we destroy our planet in thinking short term we will in essence and in turn, destroy ourselves and it could be quite painful along the way. Our foods have changed drastically, where we get it, how it grows, how we deplete our soils and weather changes and processing. Everything we need for pure health and happiness is here on earth but we must care for it carefully like we do a child and it will in return care for us. Nothing should be taken for granted, mother earth, nor our health, especially mental health.

My doctor most recently commented, you know what you are if you are hypo-manic or depressed and poor or average income, you are "crazy", you know what you are if you are hypo-manic or depressed and rich, **"eccentric"**. Money has changed our point of view even on someone with mental illness. I found this statement to be both profound and true.

MOOD

Well if you have read this far in the chapter you have now come to the best part- **MOOD**. I discovered **Evening Primrose Oil** by taking Udo's Oil in June 2011 and it seemed to mellow me a bit.
So I went to the store and talked to them about EPO, which was an ingredient in the UDO oil and I felt was important. They told me that EPO balances hormones like Estrogen- fight PMS/anger- relaxes and mellows women. It really works and I take at least 2 capsules/day after food usually.
We have so many Phyto-Estrogens in our environment- it is toxic to people, it acts like Estrogen in us- imbalances us plus our adrenals and thyroid can be out of balance (hormones) due to

them. If low thyroid, it can lead to irritability, mood swings. I have hypothyroidism and EPO is my biggest discovery- it takes away the angst and anger and allows one to be gentle, mellow and happy. A biggie!!

As well, women should take a multi mineral as well as multivitamin. **Especially trace minerals found in water or salt is important**. I got bad illnesses when I made distilled water for a few years (no minerals in it)- even tho I added minerals to it.
I sold my distiller.

HELPS ADRENALS AND STRESS HORMONES(mood):

Ashwaganda and B vitamins, Holy Basil & Rhodiola help also.

1. Ashwaganda (Indian Ginseng)- helps balance stress hormones, adrenalin in body. Nourishes and heals the adrenals. ('Innate- adrenal response', is a whole food and a good brand to try- has everything you need in it- I get mine from Finlandia)

2. B vitamins- help deal with stress (research says)- needed to calm system. Important in fibromyalgia- a Multi- B.

3. Holy Basil and Rhodiola- Help calm nerves and body too. Mellows people out. (ask nutritionist about).

4. Thyrosmart and kelp - nourishes the thyroid. regain some balance of hormones: has L-tyrosine (selenium also needed for thyroid)

5. Vitamin D- need enough Mg in body to absorb this, helps with SADS, which affects stress levels if your mood gets low.
If adrenals burn out and are exhausted, often women with too

much stress hormones have belly fat - then thyroid takes the next beating and can malfunction. Hypothyroid on the rise- obesity. Computers are actually added stress and all the coffee nowadays makes our adrenals burn out quicker.

6. Vitamin C - neutralizes cortisol (calming antioxidant) (good for skin-collagen), very vital to good health.

7. L-theanine - calms the mind (from green tea), calm your mood. Relaxes.

FATIGUE (LACK OF ENERGY)

The culprits-

>Anaemia,
>Mitral Valve Prolapse
>Wt. gain,
>Depression,
>Gluten,
>Thyroid problems,
>Insomnia (sleep problems)
>Candida Yeast Overgrowth

ANAEMIA

Often Anaemia comes with fibro. I had it. When you have Anaemia your red blood cells do not carry enough iron and thus they don't function optimally and deliver much needed oxygen to the cells of the body. You do not absorb nutrients properly in the gut to avoid Anaemia such as enough iron because often the gut will be destroyed by the gluten in your diet. **B12** (shots or sub-lingual) often assists with Anaemia as well as iron supplements (if your stomach can handle it). I find the best iron supplement right now to be 'Ultimate Iron Complex', (animal based). Take **Folic Acid** and Vitamin C as well. Vitamin C helps absorb Iron. **Iron** will help immensely with energy and clear thinking. Taking iron helps prevent hair loss.

VITAMIN B12 (plus Folic acid for nerves)

Benefits of B12 to Alzheimers and fatigue.

1. helps red blood cells- required (fatigue fighter) more o2 to cells - fight fatigue

2. youthful- helps DNA regenerate and thus replenish old dead cells , look younger, not old. Without B12 can't make new DNA

3. Nerve regeneration- require to build new nerve tissue important for brain , etc-health.
4. rid of tingling in hands and toes : Raynauds Syndrome (new nerve cells and transmission): better brain- all nerves.

We can regenerate our brain cells. Need a shot bi-monthly or sub-lingual pills. B12 helps build DNA, stress destroys it. Cannot get from food sources alot of time (B12) due to medications (they interrupt absorption), lack of other nutrients, is bound in food, unable to dissociate bond by stomach acid and thus absorb. Other factors maybe block absorption. Also our food source lacks adequate amounts. Take sub-lingual pill form, goes into blood stream right away. Can't OD (overdose) on.

I have been taking B12 since 2006/2007 in injection form, twice/month about 1 CC each time. Will keep it up now that I know the benefits. My brain has benefited tremendously from it. I was Anaemic, so docs put me on- rarely ate red meat-grass fed cattle get B12 from bacteria on the grass, no longer grass fed tho. Need Bison (wild) or organic meat to get proper B12.

.

MITRAL VALVE PROLAPSE

Often people with fibro have mitral valve prolapse (co-morbid).

The Mitral valve is the valve between the left chambers of the heart, the left atrium and left ventricle(pumper). If "prolapse", means 'leaky' a bit, sometimes requiring surgery to fix and get proper blood flow happening. Mg helps resolve this anomaly. It seems many people with fibro have this mitral valve prolapse and I feel may be in part due to Ca deposits.

WEIGHT

Extra wt is also associated with fibro as one will gain wt when one does not move so much and when you stress the fat can easily accumulate in the tummy area, this extra wt in turn also makes you more sluggish. You try carrying around an extra 50 pound backpack everyday, this is what it is like, right?......tiring. Exercise and diet will help with this as well as Mg, as it'll give you the energy you need to move.

DEPRESSION:

Depression can lead to fatigue, tiredness. I've covered alot earlier so won't go into here but know it's one of the culprits of fatigue. See Part 4 for more indepth.

GLUTEN

Fatigue also comes from Gluten I believe and it's toxicity to the body. Gluten ruins the gut.
Our ATP and mitochondria are not functioning optimally due to lack of nutrients such as Mg and trace minerals. Our blood cells do not pick up enough oxygen and circulated throughout the body well. We have no energy to exercise thus we do not create muscle and energy.

B vitamins described above help with metabolism and energy as well as cutting gluten out of your diet if you are sensitive. Mg is very important to the mitochondria of cells, the powerhouses. We do not absorb enough Mg from our diets (esp. when consuming refined carb's) nor is there adequate balance of Mg and Ca in our system.

Gluten is very much a culprit of fatigue and by cutting down or getting rid of, you will feel alot more energy!

THYROID ISSUES:

Low thyroid causes everything in the body to slow down, the heart, metabolism, digestion, etc. Thus when we have slow metabolism we feel sluggish and tired. Often people with low thyroid will have a big tummy. Thyroid controls the hormones and with low thyroid they are all out of whack, this disrupts mood, sleep and energy.
When we do not feel good emotionally we do not feel like moving much let alone exercise. Things that help low thyroid are selenium, and kale, & kelp for iodine. Kale is also good for antiplaque build up and anti-hard arteries. Chicken is good for increasing metabolism. I believe once a person comes off of gluten, the adrenals get rested and repaired and function better and this will take a burden off the thyroid thus it too can repair itself and function better. A good test to see if you are low in thyroid is a REVERSE T3 test vs. the regular T3 test.

One thing I read is that if you are borderline low thyroid and the doctor puts you on medication for it like synthroid, this will throw you into full blown hypothyroidism. It would be best if you are borderline to just supplement and assist it and then check your numbers after a period of time to see if this has helped. ....There are things like thyrosmart to assist the thyroid and also kelp (iodine).

INSOMNIA:

FOR SLEEP:

Having insomnia can make one very tired during the day.
-Almost 1/2 of people get no sleep because of a snoring partner too. So de-congest to rest- use a nedi-pot before bed or nasal strips help.
-Some can't stay asleep due to anxiety: Magnolia Bark helps reduce anxiety (like sleeping pill)- 30 mg- don't take with sleeping pills or alcohol. Take for up to 6 weeks.
-Some do not get refreshed sleep: quality is the issue not quantity. Our sleep cycle is 90 minutes long. Things to **avoid** are:
  caffeine, has a 1/2 life of 8-10 hours long.
  Alcohol, have early in night: diuretic, dehydrates, keeps you out of deep sleep.
  Tv before bed (stimulating)
  no pets in the bed (I break this rule all the time!)
  temperature: too hot or too cold hard to sleep in.

We get approx. 4-5 sleep cycles(90 min) per night.
Try to turn your brain off at night by having a worry journal, write down all your worries that night and a solution to the worry. Then tuck it away and go to sleep. Your brain will think the problems are solved.

What helps sleep is:

-Tart Cherry Juice- has melatonin in it plus antioxidants.(replace your sleeping pills with if possible)

-Passion Flower is effective in calming the brain (anxiety) before bed.

-taking warm baths before bed with Epsom salts (have Mg in), this helps relax muscles and the mind.

-Essential Oils such as lavender and/or Chamomile added to the bath assist in relaxation.

-Taking Magnesium 1/2 hour before bed helps calm the mind.

-Journal beside your bed to write down thoughts.

-A mask to shut out the light, brain will slow down in dark, light wakes it.

-Have a great pillow.
- Have a glass of water before rest, will help relax you.

-And if you have to, have about 1/2 a sleeping pill, this will help even tho addicting and not too healthy. You do need to sleep !
I feel not getting enough proper sleep is worse for you than a small sleeping pill but always check with your doctor and get their opinion.

CANDIDA YEAST OVERGROWTH:

A reason for exhaustion is Candida Yeast Overgrowth.
It is essentially an imbalance of good bacteria with fungus.
Overuse of antibiotics and increased sugar intake, increased carb's and increased alcohol consumption can all precipitate this.

Simple test to perform:
A 5 minute saliva test: in the morning spit into a glass of water (1/2 cup), if your saliva travels to the bottom and feathers up to top, means yeast; should be clear if negative for yeast.

Some symptoms are:
increased yeast infections, IBS, athletes foot, itchy scalp and skin, itchy anal area, itchy ears, bloating, mental fog, cravings, fatigue. Doctors are not traditionally trained and don't know how to treat

candida yeast overgrowth and nutrition plays a big role in flora in the intestines (balance).

Easy to manage if you have it:
Go 2 weeks:

no sugar, decrease: breads, pasta, carb's and ADD fermented foods such as saourkraut/kimchi and increase fiber- veg's. , Whole grains- brown rice, ADD probiotic supplement (25 billion and Bifido).

Some herbs that help:

1. garlic- antifungal, add to olive oil and vegs.
2. Thyme- tincture: "mouth", 1-3 ml/3x day
    or oil: apply topically- athletes foot.

In conclusion, in couple weeks exhaustion first to go away, may take couple months if alot of yeast.

So for Fatigue here are ENERGY BOOSTERS:

Here are some things that help with Energy:

-Drinks to replace coffee:
   1. Yerba Mate- like coffee but keeps you even, very healthy.
   2. Guayonlus- stimulant with L-theanine in it.
   3. Cocoa- "food of the gods" (antioxidants,
       Mg, stimulating yet calm, helps mood)

- **Astragulus-   200 mg am and pm.**

- **Brewers Yeast-** evens blood sugar as has chromium in it (sprinkle on salads)
- **Papaya juice-** Papain in it; energy
- **Brazilian Nuts-** Mg in it- energy
- **HGH-** *(Human growth hormone)*

HGH is an important one and I will discuss here briefly. HGH helps keep you young and strong. We lose it as we age as much as 85% decrease by 50. It helps keep organs healthy and muscles strong and gives you energy (like when you were young). There were injections (synthetic) that are available but recently it has been discovered that certain amino acids (4 of them) help. With these amino acids you can boost your HGH levels 600% (6 x more). You'll have faster metabolism and increased endurance.

Basically, the pituitary gland excretes HGH. This HGH helps shrink fat by using the energy for muscles. HGH increase shows in skin where it helps make you look youthful and vibrant again. As we age the pituitary gland decreases it's output, so low HGH. And thus wrinkles in the skin, lost energy as we lose up to 85% HGH when reach 50 years old.

How you get these HGH levels up safely to get the right amount for you in the body is to do the following:

1. weight resistance (lift wts. and put muscles to work)
2. get enough sleep (8 hours) :produce most HGH in first hour. Don't eat/exercise within 2 hours before bed.
3. Amino acids- 4 of them:
   i. Glycine
   ii. Ornithine
   iii. Arginine
   iv. Lysine

Amino Acids are the building blocks of Protein in the body. You can get these amino acids by eating eggs, fish, soy and some meat. However, most people need to supplement especially the older you are (over 50).

To breakdown the Amino Acids and how they help: one simple pill in an "Amino Acid Combination" of :

GLYCINE: helps build muscle, promotes good sleep, increases energy.
ORNITHINE: contributes to energy to body.
ARGININE: helps regulate blood pressure and metabolize fat.
LYSINE: turns fat food you eat into energy, good for circulation.

Use above amino's to help rebuild Human Growth Hormone.

PAIN

Everything in your body hurts, joints, muscles, even your fat!....for anyone or anything to touch you hurts. Even laying down in bed hurts. The calcium buildup in tissues causes the muscles to constantly work and contract, thus making them tired using up ATP and the gluten in the tissues causes inflammation in the joints and tissues and around organs, this hurts also. You are one sensitive beast!
It is exhausting to walk even a little , many need a cane and it hurts.

Magnesium helps block pain receptors!!

Take Mg for cramps and pain, relaxes nerve tissue, Mg helps greatly with migraines. Calms the mind, helps sleep. Pain I believe is caused by Ca buildup and toxins (gluten) in the tissues making the nerves oversensitive and hyper- reactive. Ca in tissues helps cause "ischemia" and pain, also puts nerves on high alert! Pain to touch even and all the pressure points are painful. Mg helps to BLOCK PAIN RECEPTORS on nerves, mainly how it helps I believe. Mg helps very well with migraines too. Opens blood vessels for good blood flow (helps ischemia). Mg Lowers Blood pressure.
Try to de-Calcify your tissues(there are a few products out there,

one I believe is Fulvic Acid), use Mg daily and get your gut working again to help absorb good nutrients, by getting off of gluten. A good sleep helps the body repair damage as well and settle nerves.

STATINS & Pain

Apparently Statins can contribute to muscle pain and weakness. Statins interrupt the ATP cycle and thus one should take CO Q10 with their prescription of statins so they feel less pain or tired. CoQ10 helps replace in the ATP cycle what statins block or take away.

For pain, a good product mentioned on Dr. Oz is an anti-inflammatory called ASU- Avocado, Soy bean Unsaponifiables (for osteoarthritis)
Also excellent anti-inflammatory foods are Pineapples & **Quinoa.**

ISCHEMIA & Pain

Ischemic Blood vessels, not allowing proper blood
flow (oxygen and nutrients) to tissues would explain alot about pain. Calcium and plaque buildup along with calcium constricting the blood vessels would help induce ischemia. When ischemia happens, the nerves react with pain, similar to a heart attack sensation but on a tissue, molecular level. All the nerves everywhere would light up (overreact). If one experiences ischemic blood vessels in their tiny vessels throughout the body this could in fact be a reason one feels pain and attacking of the muscles, just a theory.
There are some theories out there about the pain being sent from the Amygdala (or some major part of the brain affected by trauma) as it interprets pain incorrectly and with oversensitivity, this could be true, as the brain is connected to the rest of the whole body.

There is so much more to learn about the brain and it's affect on the body and about pain itself.

I, nor alot of experts, have any good explanation for all the pain felt in fibro patients, except that it is possibly hyperactive nerves due to exactly what , no one knows except for the above which I assume to be a good possibility; it would have to be further explored. ??

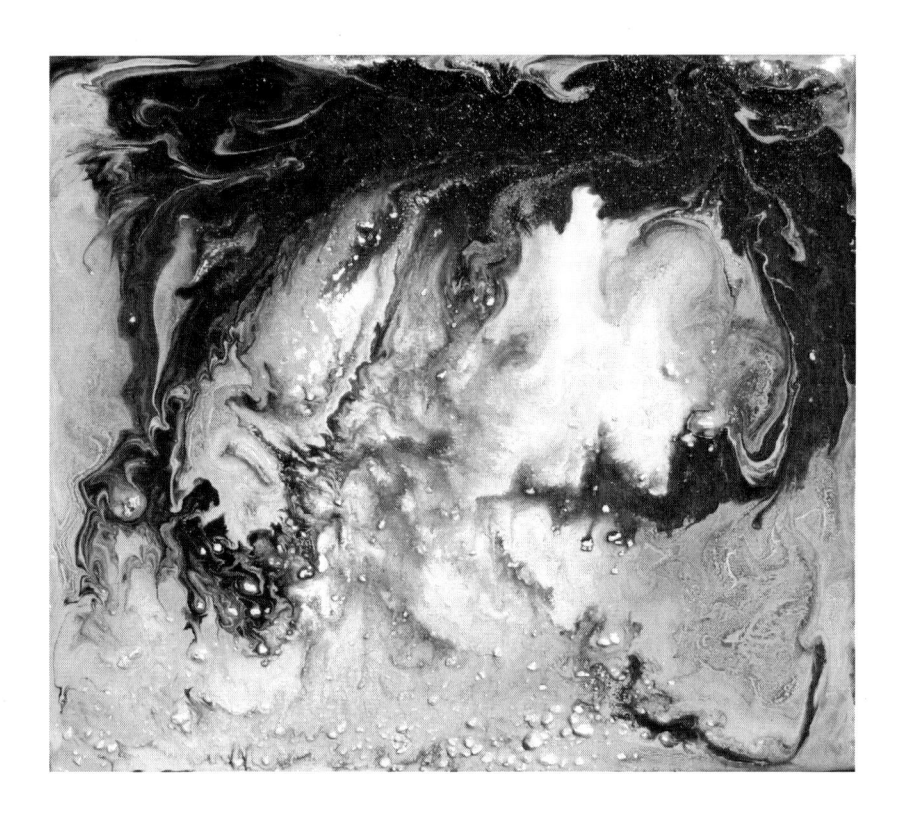

VIIII. FEELINGS/ENERGY is CONTAGIOUS

"THOUGHTS ARE FEELINGS AND FEELINGS ARE ENERGY."

Our intelligence, memories, habits and reactions form thoughts and these thoughts produce feelings which generate energy. This energy resonates at a certain frequency either high or low.

Positive energy resonates at a high frequency whereas negative very low frequency. It seems as humans we are sensitive to these frequencies on either a conscious or unconscious level, but I believe we kind of absorb them, this is why being around a happy person can lift you up and a sad person bring you down. Also why maybe friends like to be around you during the good happy times but hard to find when you are sad or need to get out of a funk. We all like to feel the high, it feels like love and a good drug. People see lows as a hard place to be in, but really it is slowing you down for a time of reflection, for you to dig up why you feel that way or have chosen to take that way. Yin and Yang (positive and negative) both exist and are necessary in life.

So it is like we have two buckets in our hearts, one filled with bad feelings and the other good feelings. We think something whether a reaction to something or somewhere (or someone) we are "stuck" on and we pick from the buckets of "love" or "Hate"(fear) -good or bad. We take this sad (bad) and it becomes energy as we feel it, it gets projected and emitted. Bad feelings emit very low energy, good feelings like love and forgiveness emit very high frequency.

So people around us whether we just stand next to them or start speaking to them pick up on the energy and frequency and it absorbs into them and they can then feel like you do. That is why it is so hard and we don't want to be around sad or angry or hurting people (say homeless) vs. a CEO (who may be passionate, motivated, energetic, healthy and on a positive high) or a priest (who is often filled with love and forgiveness). Thus moods and stress are contagious. (unless we have magnificent shields). We are all sensitive creatures and made up of energy and we reflect or absorb these energies, that is why therapists get burnt out vs. someone helping developmentally challenged children (these children often function with positive energy).

We form our thoughts which form feelings that come out as energy and where these thoughts originate is either from our intelligence (what we know), our habits (past or present) and simply reactions we may or may not be able to control. It seems people either feel joy or hurt (generalizing). Hurt comes from a thought of betrayal, fear or judgements or something deep in a person unresolved that they hang onto and reach for. It can come from a judgement of thinking the worst of someone or something

or assuming someone hurt you or by a desire to retaliate, you feel insulted and violated. Often these can be mere assumptions and not the truth so sometimes we "hurt" unnecessarily by thinking negative about something or someone. Always look for the best in others and you will always be happier, we all have two sides, light and dark, we find what we seek in others. When you look for a certain something in someone (good or bad), generally you will find it because this is where your focus is. When you focus on the best, people can express it more and all will be happy.
Don't judge, be compassionate.

Don't get "stuck" and ruminate.

A person living in the moment can easily go to feelings of joy as they are not "stuck" and they deal with "new" stuff. How they feel joy is being positive and thinking optimistically (that the present and future are good - there are good possibilities ahead), live in a place of hope vs. Fear. When one feels joy, even if based on a past memory of it (vacation or event- marry for example) they express it and people pick up on their happiness and join in. This is why at a birthday celebration people feel such happiness for the person, as they are filled with positivity and joy and love on that day, mainly remembering how much this person means and all the good times had.- joy is then emitted (a high frequency). Akin to a funeral where the main person suffering sets the tone. And people will go to an automatic place of sadness (and anger they passed or suffered and that they won't be around anymore for them)-looking into the future with fear. Rather, a funeral should be a reflection and celebration of what the person brought to the world and how they helped make it a better place (ie. where they may have helped alleviate pain, sadness and loneliness). Remember you cannot be thankful and angry at the same time! This attitude would bring feelings of appreciation and joy if people remembered all the happy times and their contribution to love. (alot of people will dwell automatically on the past whether good or bad).

Again, be optimistic and see the best in people. It is natural however, to feel sad at a funeral because we are conditioned as such, esp in N. America. We live in the future of our loss where they will be missed but rather should live in the past (good past) and present of where it has ended, but they are at peace and in a happy place (out of pain, if suffer). Tragedies are always difficult because people always go to a place of anger or resentment in their thinking that someone had malicious intent in hurting others when it was merely an accident, a mistake. Even when someone murders or injures another say out of anger or mental illness (rare), they are not in their right frame of mind and it is really an accident- a moment thing, they often regret. Mental illness is very tricky because people with mental illness are not violent for the most part unless they were violent before it came on. When people "snap" and are not in the right frame of mind they might react from a place of protection vs. outright inducing hurt. Often it will be hallucinations, voices or delusions that drive them. That a mental person would harm someone is so very rare and uncommon too as most mental people will harm themselves first before they hurt another. I say it's rare because it really is, it is just that the media (films) overreact and exacerbate that "it" was their mental illness and that all of them are evil and to be feared.

Movies and the media alike, make alot of money from scaring people and inducing fear even if they single out a certain group to blame. (The group that really bothers me is gang wars as they operate from a place of ego, power and plain vengeance, not caring who they hurt when they do- sociopaths.).

People with Mental illness suffer a great deal, they shouldn't have to also deal with the perception of fear always coming their way (low frequency energy). Alot of support and money should be going into programs, housing and research to help such people for everyone, as everyone is touched by mental illness in some capacity, even if they themselves are in denial.

The media is powerful, it conditions our thoughts and behaviour whether we wish to believe that or not. It acts like our guide or priest or teacher, and we suck in knowledge and judgements based on their theories and their dispensing information whether correct or incorrect. Media can make alot of mistakes and dispense mistruths to stories as they may only tell one side of the story.
So when we process our thoughts and feelings and turn them into energy that we release into the world, like a small child, we have to be responsible and think "do I want to infect others with negativity or positivity?" Will negativity make the situation or world a more joyful place to exist in, no not likely.
But if I don't judge and use compassion instead and forgiveness, feel just positivity (optimistic and hope) and joy and emit that, than that will infect others and maybe give them a lift as it operates at a higher frequency, and listen we all feel what others feel. That is also why it is draining and hard to be around those with problems or pain, you feel it too (unless they have a super optimistic spirit).
Often they are processing their past or habits or just a momentary reaction and cannot help emitting negativity (it often comes from fear of the worst). Mostly they are just not aware, in control and have no malicious intent (it comes from fear of pain) Humans are essentially not evil. What we do is our egos are so powerful and need to be fed because maybe we have insecurities and lack confidence or courage. We then react towards people based on feeding the ego. And this ego loves to feel strong, good and powerful, like they are "winning". So in order for it to be fed and feel this, a person will act out where they 'fight' to make their ego strong, put down others to feel powerful (I am better than you or smarter or more beautiful). This comes from insecurities and not loving yourself so you don't know how to love others. You feel punished so you must project that unto others in thinking well if I am punished so should they be. And how the ego feels good is by winning at all costs, whether it be fraudulent, being mean, cheating (not honest), hurting someone, feeling like it is a war to be won and they want to be "ahead", like a race or a game.

Bullying and Harassment are often based on the person doing it feeling insecure with themselves.

People will sometimes give you their negative energy, don't reflect it, rather instead "deflect" it, otherwise you just contribute to the problem. People naturally reflect, "mirror" each other, human nature, but we need to be self aware and control reflecting or reacting.

Alot nowadays is about money and people will virtually sell their souls to have as much as they can. Reality is we only need enough for basics, to survive but when people get money above this threshold of basics it makes them feel powerful and they get greedy and want more, thinking this is what will make them "feel" happy. And the less happy one is with themselves it 'goes', then the more money they try to have to fill their void. Money improves things, true, if used properly and for good and esp if you are giving and not selfish. People often see having money as a game, of who is winning with the most "chips", again the ego speaking. Money should be enjoyed and celebrated as a currency of exchange in getting what we need to survive and in bringing joy (like vacation memories) to your heart. If you are taking money from someone who desperately needs it or cutting their cheque short you are harming them in not having their basics and indulge a little to feel success and joy. Never let people give you a little change for something- this is petty- be generous and let it go, always think maybe they need it more than I. Appreciate the offer but turn it down out of generosity and not greedy or selfish or self-concerning. The more money you give or let go of (put out into the world) freely, it comes back in greater amounts (10x) and will serve you better, just as when you give love and it comes back. You appreciate it more and don't take it for granted.

The reason I talk about money is because **money has energy**. **Share your money and success like you would love.** Show that it has power to help. The reward is that your heart will fill with joy when you see someone eating because you shared your money which would otherwise just sit in a bank somewhere (or computer as #'s) and may even one day mean nothing or go away (currency can change). "What you give, is what you get".

Help the less fortunate, it will give you a sense of pride and help your insecurities. If you are a loving person and generous, you will automatically love yourself and feed your ego in a positive way by not "winning" but by lending a hand up the mountain of life we all climb. By doing this, you will have joy in your heart and emit a higher frequency of this energy, this is good for all and especially yourself. So when your heart feels love for a passion you do (job or hobby) or simply just appreciative of small things this emits energy and is not toxic energy like the negative is and builds up inside your body. Love is rather healing energy (why prayer works). I do not understand exactly how it helps cells function at an optimal healing level but it seems to, just as people surround someone in pain and pray and give love, they will often get better. I think Love energy trumps and dissipates hate (negative) energy as it has the higher frequency. Only a spiritual physicist might know. Just my guess. This is why if some one gives you negative energy try to deflect it with positive energy. Be nice.

If trauma happens and you can't help but feel hurt and pain and reach into your bucket of anger in your heart this energy you emit will only hurt you further as you drive people away and it builds (trapped) in your body. It will make you worse. You must yes feel it, but quickly release it and let it go for good -don't hang onto the memory of it, nor feed it like an animal or child so it remains. **FEEL, DEAL, and HEAL**. Try to deal with it as you feel it and then let yourself heal, bring in the positive. There is a blessing to everything I believe that happens to us and a good reason whether we see it at the time or not. Whether just that reason is that when we come out of our experience, we can become guides or teachers in helping others come out and heal. (**turn pain into purpose**).

The earth is a place where we all need to heal and feel this higher frequency to make it a better place to be. When one person operates at this higher frequency it impacts others to such a great degree and more powerful than negative (anger) energy. It infects others and they then feel it also and spread it. Think of it as an epidemic flu, it can just start with a few and spread like lightning across areas of the world , one continent at a time.

We are here to feel love and joy and help others feel it too (community and share). The earth is not meant to be a place filled full of pain, anger, disrespect & useless "stuff "(material things).

We all have freedom of choice- there are ultimately only two choices though- to feel anger (FEAR) or feel LOVE (joy).

When we pray for others it is also healthy for ourselves as we send out positive, healing thoughts. This can heal us at the same time and dissipate stress, inducing forgiveness which lets go of anger. Pray for your enemies- you will find peace.

Make a choice of who you want to be, walk around as an angry, hurt wounded animal (victim) or pick yourself up and love in the moment and future with optimism and love for all, including yourself. Emit positivity so you can help others feel it too, spread the "good" bug not the "bad", damaging one. This in essence will also help you as people will come around alot to be with you and feel that great feeling of joy and love. It will form a circle of support that will be there when you need it to guide you out of future pain/anger.

Sometimes we do "feel FIRST" which forms thoughts and then energy but this is rare and only with highly sensitive people, not most. One will feel the energy like when someone enters a room (say if it was Ghandi, you'd feel peace, if murderer you feel anger and despair as they emit their energies). I think this is why people like going to church, it FEELS good as people are 'behaving' and joyous.

So then we form our thoughts by 'this feeling' we get and this then will emit 'like energy ' or our own controlled energy based on our thought of the situation.

Anticipation can also bring on fear or joy, like an exam or someone walking down the aisle to marry you. This fear or joy based on anticipation will then emit an energy. We all know how calming pets are. They have no egos to fill or insecurities and operate only from a place of unconditional love and joy, emitting that energy, that is why we love our pets so. Pets are so healing, they help you emit love for them and this is healing energy for you both. Pets emit high frequency energy. Jealousy on the other hand is quite negative, don't react, protect yourself from it, consider the source- they are insecure - send love for them and yourself.

It is easy to have low frequency energy when we are exhausted. You'd notice a difference between just getting up vs. before bed. Am I right? The brain needs to be fresh and energetic to emit the higher frequency of joy (much like on a vacation when we are rested and thus full of life and optimism)

Betrayal is bad too, not sure why people betray (usually selfish or self serving motives) but try to forgive them for as Jesus would say "forgive them, for they know not what they do".

Easier said than done!

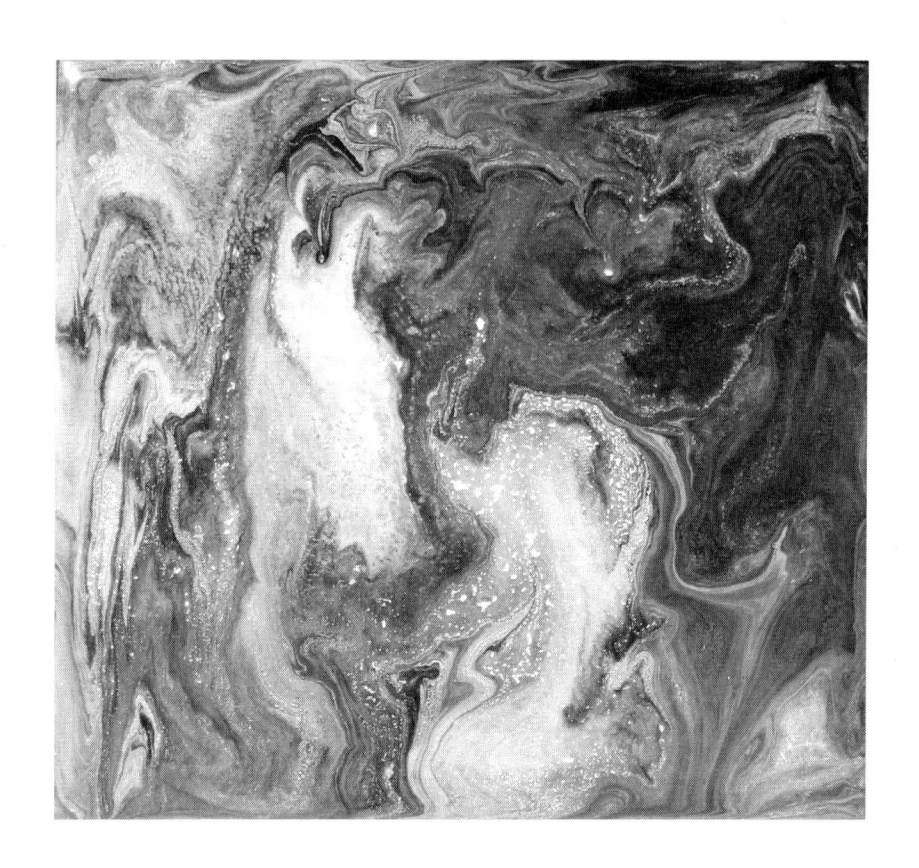

PART 3- FIBRO ELIMINATED

X. My 'prescription' (diet & costs) to help alleviate , Eliminate fibro. And pitfalls of too much Mg

(**warning**: those with kidney disorders ask their doctors before following any of the advice in this book)

Magnesium Discussed:

1. chemical rxns involved in
2. how we are so deficient and why (stress, caffeine (cortisol), gluten all deplete Mg)
3. what can lead to if deficient
4. tests to see if deficient (24 urine) and what types to take (injections best)
5. sources of ...(chlorophyll- contains Mg) VEGS.
6. Helps with ....ie. Heart and anxiety; physical and mental stuff. Musculo-skeletal issues.
7. End: what I do
8. Warnings of too much Mg

Chemical Reactions Mg involved in:

Virtually all chemical reactions in the body require enzyme systems to help the biochemical reaction take place. Enzyme systems consist of 3 parts generally:
1. a specific protein molecule
2. another smaller organic compound (often a vitamin ie. Vit b6)
3. a charged mineral (zinc, copper, manganese or magnesium)

"Magnesium is a critical co-factor in more then 300 enzymatic reactions in the human body"

Potassium (a univalent cation- electrical charge of +1) and Magnesium (divalent cation- electrical charge of +2) are the most abundant cations within cells of the body. Magnesium is the number 1 most abundant divalent cation.

There are over 200 published chemical studies as of 1996 documenting the need for Magnesium.

Magnesium is extremely important in cardiovascular health.

Mg helps :
- **Block pain receptors**
- **Calm overactive nerves**
- **Calm the mind**
- **Create energy** (important to mitochondria (**ATP**))

Mg helps de-stress- helps adrenals and thyroid (hormones), maybe block adrenaline/cortisol and help the Amygdala (in overdrive) "How it does" is not as important as the fact "it does". We'll leave it to the scientists to investigate and reveal.
Mostly obstetricians use injectable magnesium sulfate for the treatment of high blood pressure and pre-clampsia and eclampsia of pregnancy. But now, conventional physicians in the US are using magnesium to treat patients with Acute heart attacks, chronic cardiovascular disease, heart arrhythmias, diabetes, asthma, CFS and many other disorders.

How we are so deficient and why:

We used to be alot calmer before gluten (say in the early 1900's) and new farming practices where now soils are depleted. The fact gluten is depleted of magnesium (over processed) and a ruined intestine leads to low absorption of required nutrients such as magnesium to help keep the body and mind calm. It is no wonder with hype of coffee now also that we are so stressed out and irritable to bout (too much cortisol and adrenaline). Magnesium is no longer in our water sources either as it is de-mineralized, one must drink mineral water to get mineral benefits. At least 40% of Americans are deficient when it comes to Magnesium.

What lead to if deficient:

Symptoms of magnesium deficiency can affect virtually every organ system of the body namely skeletal muscle, leading to twitches, cramps, muscle tension, muscle soreness (back aches, neck pain, tension headaches and TMJ).

Also **Cardiovascularly** one may experience chest tightness or the sense of not being able to take a deep breath. One can experience:

-**impaired contraction of smooth muscles** (ie. urinary spasms, menstrual cramps, constipation)

-**photophobia** (sensitive to oncoming bright headlights)

-**loud noise sensitivity**(due to stapedius muscle tension in ear)

The **Central nervous system** is affected with Mg deficiency, symptoms will include:

- insomnia
- anxiety
- hyperactivity and restlessness with constant movement
- panic attacks
- agoraphobia
- PMS

Peripheral nervous system symptoms are:

- numbness, tingling & vibratory sensations.(ie. Raynauds)

Cardiovascular systems symptoms include:

- palpitations
- heart arrhythmias
- angina (due to spasms of the coronary arteries)
- high Blood pressure
- mitral valve prolapse

People with Mg deficiency often seem to be "uptight". Other general symptoms include:

– salt cravings
– both carbohydrate craving and carb intolerance
– breast tenderness

Test to take to see if deficient: (24 hour urine test)

Lab testing is of limited value since Mg is found primarily "in cells", thus the serum magnesium may be normal in spite of a significant Mg deficiency. Red blood cell Mg test is a little better. Optimally tho, is the "**Mg loading test**". In this test, a patient collects a 24 hour urine sample and total Mg is measured, patient then given an injection of a specified amount of Mg and another 24 hour urine specimen is collected. Mg is again measured. It is concluded there is Mg deficiency if the body retains more than a certain amount of Mg, holding onto the Mg that has been injected. Perhaps the best method of diagnosing Mg deficiency, is however the combination of signs and symptoms of Mg deficiency, which improves with a therapeutic dose of either oral or injected Mg.

Some Mg sources:

One can get some Mg from food in the diet if the body (gut) is able to absorb it. Eat a variety of whole foods, whole grains, nuts, seeds, and vegetables, preferably grown on naturally composted soil. The green colour of green vegetables is due to it's chlorophyll, which is a molecule that contains magnesium. So green is good! Avoid anything with white sugar and white flour in them as most Mg is removed from them.

How to take Mg (types):
There are oral Mg supplements or an injection. Magnesium is available in many forms. Cheapest is Mg oxide, but not absorbed as well as other forms like chelated Mg, Mg glycinate or Mg aspartate. Prescription form of Mg chloride, known as "Slow-Mag" has been used successfully with alot of patients. Mg Taurate, an unusual form of Mg is Mg chemically combined with amino acid derivative Taurine and is effective as Taurine has a calming effect on the nervous system like Mg. It helps strengthen the heart muscle too. The two being synergistic together are helpful with all forms of cardiac and nervous system disorders. I myself am happy so far with Mg glycinate (or bis-glycinate) Finlandia is where I get mine, they produce it under their label.

Dose: the RDA for Mg is 350-400 mg "elemental"Mg. One must watch the 'total amount' of a capsule as it may be 400 mg with the

elemental Mg in it only 100 mg of total. So you must take 4 capsules to get the 400 mg elemental Mg. (the capsules total 400 mg refers to the "amino acid complex" that is bound to the Mg). Most people may only take one- two capsules per day which means they are well below the RDA (recommended dietary allowance).
A therapeutic does is roughly 400- 1000 mg daily of elemental Mg in divided doses. In people with normal healthy kidneys, it is difficult to reach toxic levels of Mg. However, too much oral Mg may result in diarrhea.

Beware *patients suffering from chronic kidney failure as their kidneys have difficulty eliminating Mg and a toxic buildup may occur. If so, toxic levels may lead to a severe depression of the entire nervous system, even coma and death. So please beware. This is however, extraordinarily rare but I feel very worth mentioning. It occurs only in patients with severe kidney function impairment.*

In general, Mg doses of 1000 mg/day or less is very safe. It is mainly water soluble and your body will just rid of the excess it doesn't need or use. (It is also a good idea to take it with some calcium- for balance.)

Mg Sources:

Mg is crucial to more than 300 bodily functions- many of which give you energy.
some Mg containing foods are:

-chocolate (mainly dark)
-bananas
-kidney beans
-black beans
-whole wheat bread (will have gluten)

-brown rice
-lentils
-oatmeal (may have gluten?)
-quinoa
-raisan Bran (may have gluten)
-spinach
-shredded wheat (gluten)
need approx. 5 servings/day

-3/4 of Americans are Mg deficient
-are you irritable, tired, weak? ....if so read on,

<u>What Mg helps with</u>:

Helps with **Heart** and **anxiety, physical and mental**, and **musculo-skeletal** issues.

Oral Mg supplementation may be helpful to a wide variety of medical disorders (besides fibro) they are:
- high blood pressure
- asthma
- angina pectoris
- CAD
- Cardiac arrhythmias
- CFS/fibro
- all types of musculo-skeletal disorders (ie. Rheumatoid arthritis)
- Epilepsy
- Mitral valve prolapse
- ED (erectile dysfunction)
- Diabetes
- Parkinsons
- Alzheimers
- MS (?)
- anxiety; panic disorders

and many other medical and psychiatric conditions.

Surprisingly, Mg is given for acute heart attacks. Given by either intramuscular injection or as an intravenous drip. Studies show it reduces the death rate and complications of acute heart attack victims. Those suffering from CFS also seem to do better with Mg given by injection studies have shown. This may be due to the superior absorption of injectable Mg or because high concentrations in the body are necessary for maximal therapeutic effects. Injectable Mg is often found in some EDTA chelation therapies. (Naturopaths do)

(Magnesium exists in many combinations, magnesium glycinate/ bisglycinate (these are the very best), magnesium citrate, magnesium chloride, etc., The form I most like and have less bowel problems with is the 'magnesium glycinate', it seems most gentle while potent. You can take alot of it in that form without the diarrhea I found for myself, you may too.(and I am sensitive)

how much to take:

RDA (recommended daily allowance) is 350 elemental Mg daily, so around 4-5 tablets of 500 mg 'total' Magnesium- look for the breakdown, usually a 500mg capsule will have 100 mg elemental Mg.

I take min 300 elemental Mg daily now, but sometimes just periodically when I feel I need it most. Helps with absorption of B vitamins and Vit D, two other very important vitamins to have in your system.

I took 2 grams (2000 mg : 4- 500 mg tablets) for approx. 2 weeks then 1 gram (1000 mg- 2 - 500 mg tablets) for few months til better then 500 mg/day (maintenance, just when feel low, cramps or achey). I hardly take at all anymore tho I will start taking a maintenance level soon again after I know how Gluten Elimination is affecting Fibro.

MY DIET: (and WHAT I DO)

80-90% Gluten free diet
Veg Powder 1 tsp per day (get everything)- in Smoothie
Vit B's (for stress)
EPO (for mood- balance hormones, no PMS)
Mg (calm, relax, sleep, lower Blood Pressure)
Vit D (good for SADS, depression, anxiety, overall health)
Vit B12 (every 2 weeks 1 ml) (for brain health)
Multivitamin (good quality- SISU) every couple days
Water- lots of filtered water (min 1 L/day)
Fresh fruit and Vegs
Himilayan salt and fresh ground pepper used only (no table salt)
Yogurt almost daily (dairy tho)
Protein, like eggs and chicken (the odd beef)
REST (nap when can)
Meditation (2 X /day)
Yoga when can (at least 1/week- grounding, breathing)
Exercise when can 10-30 min 3X/week
limit email and computer time
limit tv intake, limit news (often too negative)
Pet- have pet if can
Friend to call
Baths – at least 1/day, with lavender or epsom salt when have
Say Prayer of "THANKS" before sleep, reflect on day a bit
Coffee 2x/day
avoid gossip or negative energy
Hobby- create, write, paint, read, swim
Journal- have a journal (your best friend!)

"practice Spontaneous Kindness"
drive calmly
listen to music everyday (upbeat, positive), read the odd time
eat chocolate 1/ week (good source of Mg)
watch Dr. Oz (but take with grain of salt- entertainment) 2x/wk
take Sunday for self "OFF"- me time- naps, whatever.

Other vitamins I will take:

*Adrenal support : INNATE brand (took alot in beginning of healing)
chromium picolinate (manages blood sugars)
kelp (helps thyroid- iodine)
L-Arginine (helps with blood vessels- arteries, open)
L-Tyrosine (helps with stress)
Ashwaghanda (helps with stress and adrenals)
ZINC (helps brain)
Rhodiola (adrenals and stress)
L-Theanine (calms while making you alert)- in green tea
Oil of Oregano (for colds & flu- drops under tongue)
visit health food store approx 1/month to discuss things, get latest.
Green powders & Whey Protein Powder (if not vegan)

COST (according to 2014/2015- approx., may vary)

Veg Powder : 15- 25 $/month (Whole Foods- "green vibrance" brand) or a $35 bucket of 'greens'.
Vit B's 5$/month (Most vitamins from Finlandia or Whole Foods)
*Mg: 20$/month (Mg glycinate, best on bowels- Finlandia brand)
*Fish Oil : 8-10$/month (I like liquid & refrigerate)
*EPO : 20$/month (I like Natural Factors EPO- evening primrose oil)
Quality Multivitamin: 10$/month (SISU- sometimes has B already in)
*Vit D : 3-4 $/month (SISU- Vit D3)

B12: 3$/month (injections or sublingual tablets (under tongue))
Filtered Water : Filter 3$/month (36$ for one year, put right on tap (BRITA)

---

*APPROXIMATELY 85-100 $/MONTH TOTAL for basics. (most Important is EPO, Mg and Vit D : 42$/month) If only have 20$ get the Mg and stay off gluten. (lots of water & meditate, is free)

*FINANCIALLY IMPORTANT HERE: can try to get a 'Monthly Nutritional Allowance' if on disability, one of my friends has, it pays about 100-200$/month extra for Nutritional Supplements/month- try get your family doctor to fill out the form and explain.

So Easy Steps (Resolve):

1. MAGNESIUM: take, blocks pain receptors on nerves, gives energy, calming, min 350- 400 mg elemental Magnesium/day (RDA) (for first week I took 500-600 elemental mg/day to rid pain),
many forms- you may get injections from your doctor, already discussed importance. Mg needed to absorb Vitamin D and Vit B's. Get in Epsom salt baths (magnesium sulfate) for muscle pain too and just relaxing, letting stress go.

2. GET VITAMIN D: (min 2000 IU/day- morning) helps with SADS which alot of people in Vancouver get (or use a medical light for it, helps too). More studies are confirming Vit D importance to health.

3.   TAKE VITAMIN B's : helpful with stress & required for overall health.

4.   GET OFF GLUTEN: imperative to getting nutrients you put into your gut and clearing up inflammation which causes pain and fatigue, may take couple months to get better intestines, to a full years time. Wean yourself off it or just go cold turkey but gluten is addictive so expect some withdrawal symptoms. Remember 70% of immunity is in the GUT!! As well where we make 90% of our Serotonin.

5.   EPO : (Evening Primrose Oil) for mood stabilizing (hormones for women, especially good for PMS). Makes you happy actually and very calm and cool.

6.   VEGETABLE POWDER: to get Energy, Mg and nutrients, this I found made me even better with clear thinking and my intestines were healthy enough to benefit . Feel alot happier in mood too taking it. What to look for in a good one: no fillers, minimal processing plus probiotics. I like the one I use, called "Green Vibrance" (is gluten free and has probiotics in it). About 31$ - for one month or more supply.

7.   THINKING HABITS: change them to hope and optimism, positivity, MEDITATE, set goals, take steps everyday to reach them. Help others. Share. Give thanks everyday for what you do have in life. When you meditate, feed yourself good and healthy thoughts, ones that move you ahead (forward) in life, not backwards or stuck. Meditation has proven benefits, make the time. **We ARE what we THINK!**

8.   EXERCISE OR YOGA: if you can. DO at least 3x/week. Take Walks. Helps endorphins in brain and overall muscle and body function. Benefits both mental and physical healing.

9. TAKE CARE OF YOUR ADRENALS: they just may be burned out due to stress (more than likely). So take herbal support for, see a nutritionist. I like Ashwaghanda and Rhodiola, in INNATE Brand, a whole food (not alot of processing). Have to watch processing and fillers in supplements.

10. TAKE A QUALITY MULTI-VITAMIN EVERY DAY OR COUPLE DAYS (I like SISU personally they have high quality and in capsule, not hard tablet form). These will work better when your gut is healed.

11. *DRINK PLENTY OF WATER: to flush out toxins and help rid inflammation.

Fibro is very much both a mental and physical ailment therefore you have to tie them together and work on the health of them both at the SAME time. Mind, Body and Spirit all affect each other as all are tied as ONE.

The above steps helped Eliminate my fibromyalgia within a couple weeks the pain disappearing, to 2-6 months where I feel none of the symptoms and never felt better. So I can imagine in a year my body may be completely rejuvenated and healed.
I sure hope the above steps work for you and you found information worthwhile in this book that I have shared, I may only be a trial of one but I have tried many other things to no avail and this way is just so simple, Mg is Magic!

STORYBOARD: tell your story.
　　　If you find positive results or end up being better like me, I would love for you to **share your experience** and if this book helped you.
If you go to the FIBROSUCCESS.COM website and log in your story (short is good or long) on the storyboard, it will inspire others who are skeptical or not quite sure and need help. Maybe your methods will help them instead? Good luck and good health!

AS WELL WHAT I DO:

baths daily, sometimes with epsom salts
hydrate with water: 1 L/day or 4-6 glasses daily, filtered or mineral water (flushes toxins out of body)
Use himalayan salt in food with fresh ground pepper (trace mineral- our bodies do need GOOD salt, like sea salt)
Use real butter (no substitutes)
drink mineral water at times (gerolsteiner)
Exercise when can, 1-3 km on treadmill or a yoga class

VITAMINS: (* means religiously)
Multivitamin ~ every 2-3 days
*Evening Primrose Oil (mood)
Magnesium Glycinate (energy, relaxation) only when needed now
*B vitamins (for stress - we all have) (take with Mg)
*Vit D 2000-3000/day (for whole body: mood/SADS -seasonal affective disorder)
Vit C (some at times- good for skin, cortisol levels, etc)
Zinc (for brain and immunity)
*Omega 3's- fish oil: 1 tsp/day (brain)
*B12 ; usually injections 2 x /month (brain and iron-energy too)
'Innate Adrenal Response' (ashwaghanda- supports exhausted adrenals)
Kelp (Mg and iodine) sometimes to help thyroid (iodine)
Arginine sometimes (helps blood vessels)
chromium picolinate sometimes (helps level blood sugars; reduce wt.)
iron- "ultimate iron complex"
Brewers Yeast- helps reduce bad cholesterol

DIET AND MEALS:
Breakfast: Dr. Oz Green Drink or my smoothie for breakfast every day with 2 eggs with odd bacon or hash browns or just Fruit /yogurt

Lunch: lentil soup (amy's-gluten free) or chicken or salad
Dinner: rice pasta with meat (protein) /salad at times; veg stir fry/ wheat free pizza/salmon with cauliflower
** throughout day will do 1/3 carb's, 1/3 protein, 1/3 vegetables (snack: nuts(vit E), popcorn)
Dessert: bowl of fruit/ice cream - desserts in wheat belly
coffee intake: try to limit to 2-3 cups /day or less, will need less as less gluten in diet and more energy in body.
The time of day I eat most is 2-4 pm, not much after 7 pm. Eat good yogurt (olympic, activia) almost daily.

Dr. Oz's green drink:
spinach
kale
mint
pineapple/pineapple juice
apple or apple juice (not too much due to sugar content)
celery
cucumber
ginger
lemon juice and lime juice
carrots or carrot juice
berries when have- raspberry, blueberry, blackberries
parsley
couple slices of orange
blend in mixer all together, add some ice cubes to taste better!
(may add some almond milk, banana, yogurt or protein powder)

<u>MY SMOOTHIE</u>: (is delicious and sweet)
1   cup yogurt (usually strawberry or vanilla)
1.5   cups almond milk (usually vanilla)
3/4   cup blueberries
1/2   orange
 1/2   apple
  5-6   ice cubes

1 scoop green VEG powder (+ 1 scoop protein powder at times)

(Blend in blender for approx. 30 seconds- makes 2 cups, I put one in the fridge for later)

WHAT I RECOMMEND:

Take Mg glycinate 2-3 grams per day for one to two weeks to rid of body pain, then take gluten out of diet (gradual or cold turkey), introduce multivitamins and gluten free products into diet with Omega 3 oils (use EPO for mood, will help alot with irritability) use Mg glycinate when needed for energy and to rid of pain when eat something gluten by accident or just for a pick me up.
detoxify Ca out of tissues with Fulvic acid or the like (ask nutritionist- be careful with)

Exercise when can as helps with muscles regeneration and wt loss (burn off your belly)- and get serotonin production in brain.
take some Mg (500 mg) before bed as will rest mind and calm body-sleep better. wake better.
aside: Sulfur helps heal skin so may with gut, try taking some organic stuff maybe, will help clear acne and scars I believe(?)
note: *Silica helps alot with hair and skin being healthy looking.

Omega 3's

Omega 3's help
        stabilize hormone levels
        reduce inflammation, help joints
        helps brain function
        helps Cardiovascular health (American Heart Association claims)

WHAT TO LOOK FOR IN AN OMEGA 3

-potency --- mg, at least 1000 mg in omega 3 , not just 1000mg in fish oil.

- enteric coated ---so mass pass into the intestine where absorbed

-added Vit D ---a vit D deficiency has been linked to silent inflammation

-purity ---get certified "IFOS" -international fish oil standard

IF YOU DO THE ABOVE, you will feel immediate pain relief in one to two weeks if not days (and energy) and in 6-12 months feel completely relieved of fibro symptoms, post gluten riddance. Your hair will grow back, you will lose wt,, you will get lots done, brain fog disappears, your skin will improve, you will just feel a whole lot better. Plus you will sleep better and not be depressed or moody. (fingers crossed).

Resolve: (conclusion)
(how to resolve)

So essentially due to being a women and having low testosterone and high Estrogen, (plus high stress), you have more/bigger stressors and thus more cortisol and adrenalin. This triggers the brain into fight or flight, affecting mainly the Amygdala and Limbic systems in the brain. This in affect exhausts the adrenals (will get resultant hormone imbalance). So with adrenals breaking down this affects hormones more (thyroid gland affected), pulls them all out of balance. This hormonal balance is very important for both the mind and body to function. (Researchers are just beginning to discover how hormones affect the brain to such a great degree.) We get irritable, moods and exhausted with improper hormone balance.

We collect Calcium in our tissues (partly due to hormone imbalance).
Ca needs a certain amount of Mg in the body to stay liquified and go where it is suppose to, if not, it collects in tissues and joints and the heart. This important Mg is not avail because it is not in our diet and/or our gut is too destroyed to absorb it efficiently. Ca in our tissues causes plaques, contraction and ischemia of our small blood vessels. Thus vessels are not open enough for tissues and muscles to receive much needed blood, O2 and nutrients to work. Our nerves are thus on high alert- we get pain all over. Our gut is sensitive to gluten and thus destroyed (maybe leaky gut syndrome)- Mg is not absorbed along with other nutrients. So we cannot balance out or rid of extra Ca – it collects in tissues making us weak and rigid. (and old).

The body reacts to leaky gut or gluten as an allergen and becomes inflamed, this causes pain (histamines?) and fatigue as your body is always in attack mode. SO body is attacking itself and the mind is simultaneously under attack with constant fight or flight. How do you stop all this you ask? ....My body is breaking down.... and it will with the weakest organs (by genetics) being attacked and destroyed first.
Fibro can be genetic in this regard due to our cells structure and function, our allergies, sensitivities and our behaviour (personality- how we respond to and deal with stress). They are all linked and depending how and where one lives they may fall victim while others in their family don't.

So here are my methods and steps to heal:

1. Take Mg- will calm the mind and stop the Amygdala and Limbic system from being in overdrive. This calming will stop all

the cortisol and adrenalin and give the adrenals needed rest. The thyroid will thus rest too and hormones will balance better. (take Vitamin C to neutralize cortisol too)

2. Take EPO to assist with all the irritability til your hormones are better balanced. With adrenals resting and repairing, this will improve you eventually physically. Assist adrenals with Ashwaghanda mix too. So with the mind and adrenals resting, the Mg will also open blood vessels to muscles and tissues and eradicate the ischemia causing pain,etc. Mg works to block pain receptors too so pain will soon go away. Energy will come too as Mg is vital to ATP (cell power). You will feel calm, energetic, less pain and healthier (stronger). You will sleep better too. (as the mind gets calmed) Sleep is imperative to healing very much so, we all need the downtime to repair. (attack on mind calmed- vit B helps with this too)

3. Now with that all under control, take GLUTEN or an "allergen" **OUT** of your life (diet or environmental). Removing gluten will help heal your gut, stop the inflammation (attack on body) and in repairing will better absorb nutrients it needs, you will get Mg, Vit D, Vit B, etc. With reduced inflammation, your pain again will dissipate. You will automatically feel more energy as your body is no longer attacking "something" or itself. Fatigue will go away. Mg will be absorbed, serotonin will be made (90% from gut) this will help the depression-serotonin not proven (the latest) to impact depression tho. So the gut is healing and will take about one year. Once you remove allergens, histamines will stop too (do these cause pain and fatigue?)

Your body will physically come into "balance" and your diet will now be beneficial to the body. While doing all things above, practice positive thinking and optimism and planning (meditate). Feed your mind healthy, good thoughts, I talk alot about depression, our thinking which we CAN control plays into depression a great deal, it will determine often if we stay stuck in

it or get out and heal. With fibro often people are so deep in the illness they cannot see the forest for the tress and have no focus outside of themselves. (how the brain is, in fog)
So mind, body and spirit all healing together, and eventually nutrients will be absorbed. You will notice hair growth which proves the nutrients are being absorbed and utilized and blood flow is taking place. Soon you will be able to exercise, little by little, this will also create energy, increases circulation and detox's the body. Flush the body constantly with GOOD WATER, as you heal to flush out toxins and excess garbage that has collected in the body. I have used products to de-calcify my body and feel they work but this step is extreme and you may want consultation due to removing too much or how. I feel that Ca is trapped in the tissues and as the body will eventually flush them out I found that things like Fulvic acid (decalcifier) assisted greatly.

It is when we get Ca trapped in our tissues where it should not be that we age, feel old and rigid and are inflexible and lack energy. The contraction it causes will cause fatigue and pain. And most recently, also it has been proven that too much Ca leads to HEART DISEASE especially for women. It collects in the heart and arteries and causes hardening of the arteries and added plaque. A hard heart is not good. It is suppose to be a flexible pumping muscle after all.

SO eventually you will feel calm, happy, energetic, pain free, able to work again and exercise, will sleep (even with a little sleeping pill), you will last the whole day and get things accomplished in your life as well as be able to "show up" for yourself and others in life! You will become a powerhouse and feel younger and stronger. You will have learned how to handle stress better so you do not exhaust your adrenals again and as well now you will have mind body, spirit balance in your life. You have learned alot about yourself thru your journey, take that with you moving forward. You can now make goals and dream again! You will be healthy and happy, this is my hope for you.

I feel at least 50% to 75% of all fibro patients are nutrient deficient and this leads to this illness (weakening of the body) and that once the gut and mind are running optimally, it can be "beat" (cured), so I feel quite strongly that this book, while not helping all, will help several/many people, I hope one of them is you. Good luck and good health.

Any questions, testimonials, stories and opinions etc, please go to my website FIBROSUCCESS.COM and ask or blog!

Even the title "fibrosuccess" is all about positivity!

Stay positive and you will get better!

WARNING OF TAKING TOO MUCH Mg

Mg supplementation should be AVOIDED with severe **kidney problems** (severe renal insufficiency when on dialysis) and also with **Myasthenia Gravis.**

Use caution if you have severe adrenal weakness or low blood pressure. If one consumes too much Mg, this can cause muscle weakness, if this occurs just use more calcium temporarily to relieve. *Signs and symptoms of too much Mg (hypermagnesia)* can be similar to magnesium deficiency and include: changes in mental status, diarrhoea (dehydration), nausea, appetite loss, muscle weakness, difficulty breathing, extremely low blood pressure, dizziness, and irregular heartbeat.

Just because your body rids Mg as it is water soluble does not mean that excessive amounts over time cannot be somewhat harmful, if you feel you are encountering a problem please seek medical attention or take the high doses of Mg UNDER the care of a Professional who can monitor any side effects of high dose Mg. Just be aware that most doctors, especially western won't be agreeable with this method and may fight you on it because of either lack of knowledge or the safety concerns mentioned above pending your individual situation or case. If they truly fight you on it and you feel strongly about trying it, I suggest to just try a high dose for maybe one week only and see if you notice a difference. Just please be aware of how you feel and any negative changes as everyone reacts differently and just because I did not have problems doesn't mean you won't necessarily. And just because it is natural does not mean it cannot be toxic to the body or not cause problems. Take this with caution. Journal how you feel if you like and show your doctor. I am rather against high doses for a prolonged period of time like more than 6 months.

The best is to try to decrease the Ca levels in your tissues and use a maintenance level of Mg or a balance of Mg and Ca long term.

CONCLUSION:

Fibro is such a mystery to most, what I present is tried and true for myself after alot of other methods and struggles, it is thru my hard work and time and paying attention to what works and finding out why and how, that I have come to write this book. I might be way off but I may be RIGHT ON, you be the judge, it takes minimal time, effort and cash to try my methods and my only hope is to help just one person so maybe that is you? Maybe after reading this book and trying, and if it works, you can pass the book onto your family doctor and help educate them with this worthy point of view of fibromyalgia, the mystery alot of people don't believe in. Well I know it exists and while you will always have those small few who take advantage and maybe fake it to get something, alot of people genuinely suffer and must be helped to have a healthier life and fulfilment and be out of pain. I believe I have just 'connected all the dots' here and I really hope people will find it beneficial in their lives, it took me over 2 years to write and I did it in longhand first, so alot of work but a nice journey and good process I have enjoyed. I love to help others if I am truly able and they want to truly help themselves.

I feel it is a combination of contributing factors and all must be resolved:
1. Mg deficient
2. Gluten/ inflammation
3. The Amygdala
4. Ca in tissues due to low Mg
5. Adrenal burnout/ thyroid issues
6. stress/trauma

My book covers all these.

Follow my simple steps and hopefully you too will regain your life and footing and also contribute. Above all, Be PATIENT and try to figure out what works for you individually as we are all individuals, alot of problems do exist I believe because of poor diets though.

Unfortunately we live in such a 'convenient' world in this day that we don't take time for proper nutrition (nor do some farmers) on which our bodies are based, along with our thoughts. Remember thoughts are powerful, they feed us too and mold who we are and who we become. Get rid of old patterns or bad habits, form new healthy ones, only you can truly help yourself. Start today!

"The Hardest part of doing something , is finishing it!" (jemma)

"The only 'failure' that exists, is in NOT TRYING."

"The difficult part is not in letting go but learning to start over."

"Dream Lofty dreams, for thoughts become things"

"Luck is on your side, you just have to work for it." (jemma)

"It is not losing, but is freedom"

"Everyone is Lucky, ...few are prepared".

"Be like the grasshopper, go with the ebb and flow of life, for we do not know our destiny" (jemma)

"What we think today, tomorrow will bring " (jemma)

"The more I endure, the better I get at enduring it!" (jemma)

"One cannot be pitiful and powerful at the same time"

"Your past does not define you, it prepares you"

"You cannot teach someone who is unwilling to learn"

SOME CONCLUDING THOUGHTS TO GO WITH THE SUMMARY DIAGRAM:

DIET
vital to health- most important what we put on and IN our bodies (toxins and GMO'd) Vitamins and minerals essential for good health (need to supplement - our food system and soils have changed drastically)
Gut Health- Immunity is key to strength and fight disease (illness)- once you fix your tummy, your genes and thus body will be able to run optimally. I believe a healthy gut may even help resolve Crohn's disease (?)

HORMONE AND BRAIN (interrelated)

EPO- mood- brain injury, concussions, PTH (parathyroid hormone)

Sometimes when one has a Brain Injury- mood disorder can result and suicides. Changes Brain function, structure and chemistry. Hormones and brain are intimately connected as is Testosterone and Estrogen especially. Probably connected to limbic system (emotion centre) and prefrontal cortex (reasoning) and Amygdala (fight or flight).
Mood- balance Hormones to help mood and Brain ----EPO (Evening Primrose Oil) balances at least Estrogen. What also helps is Omega 3's, Mg+ and Vit D (SADS), folate and zinc (not too much of this one).

We need Omega 3's oils for the brain. Mg is needed to make Hormones (adrenals and thyroid are Hormone centers and tied together)- with all the biochemical reactions they are involved in. **Thus Brain needs Hormones, so needs Mg**, this helps mood (calming) and then once you have hormone production, use EPO to balance these hormones- mood evens. **Need Mg to absorb Vit**

D and B vits. Vit D proven to be so important but can't absorb it without enough Mg.
Women more prone to hormone imbalances, why so moody vs. men. Women are quicker (and more prone) to burn out their adrenal glands and this then affects the thyroid, in which both then affect hormone production and the Brain. **Mg will help make these hormones**. But you must remove refined and processed food from your diet as these products will absorb Mg and carry it out of the body (also lacks Mg in first place too)

So women more prone to hormone imbalances is also due to structurally different brains and hormones in the body. Nutrition affects hormones and also what we get from our environment (phytoestrogens, BPA's, pesticides, etc), so goes back to how important diet is.

It is just found in research that at different times of the month (menstrual cycle) there are dopamine spikes in the prefrontal cortex. This may help explain PMS and we can now see how intimately hormones affect brain function. We have a long ways to go in studying hormones and the brain together. A long ways. I think we actually take it for granted how involved in each other they really are.

Thus I would conclude that hormones and physicality of the brain may play a role in structuring "our thoughts", as when not so healthy, we tend to think more negative and this negativity then impacts it further and worse and worse it gets (cycle). They work together and impact each other but I feel if you were to pick one, the physical impacts the mental more (like lack of proper nutrients, a persons personality-genes) but then it can also be stated that when we have trauma (which affects us mentally/emotionally) this can break the mind physically (injure the precious Amygdala) so in this case it was the emotional mind that caused the physicality to not work, again tied so intimately together, I think one cannot separate the two.

WHY WOMEN HEART DISEASE ON THE RISE

estrogen --> Ca --> hard arteries ---> heart attacks, pain, fatigue

(why we should not give women estrogen in menopause, it leads to Ca deposits is my guess) women especially during menopause take extra Ca as told by their doctor and everyone to.

Women encouraged past 20 years to take more Ca when Mg going down in intake and ratios very off balance. Osteoporosis is not greatly helped by this assumed hypothesis and it is rather now realized Mg intake just as important to bone health. It was thought just Ca alone is important in bones just because we have our greatest stores of Ca in bones. But really it is Ca, Mg and Phosphorous "together" that save bone loss and these ratios in balance is very important. Not too much of one or throws off others. Have seesaw balance.

So this assumed hypothesis of requiring Ca in diet is just as 'they' said whole grains bread is good... "trendy theories". And our food and where it comes from has changed and been altered too much (GMO'd) for these theories to hold any value or truth. Consuming too much of either of these leads to huge immunity (gut) problems and heart disease, etc.

Affects weight a great deal which is negative on the body's functioning. Mg helps keep Ca fluid in the body and put into bones. If not enough Mg, Ca^{++} will be deposited in places in the body if not put back into bones and often this will be plaques in arteries and lead to hardening, constrictions and heart attacks.

Inflammation in the arteries I feel open the door for Ca^{++} to collect on/in certain spots where arteries are inflamed or injured, along with cholesterol. Just my theory, there are theories that exist that say sugar causes injury to blood vessels, this could also open the door for Ca^{++} to collect there.

Ca++ causes contraction too throughout the body, thus contracts the vessels when they should be open and relaxed and flexible for proper blood flow to deliver nutrients and thus no pain.

STRESS AND GREY HAIR

We get grey hair because of stress (most reason or genetics)--- Stress destroys the hair follicles (melatonin production) and the DNA of the brain--> this is why as we age, so does our brain, we get depressed, go crazy, senile, alzheimers- the more stress, the quicker and more severe the decline. (Zinc helps a bit).

SUMMARY DIAGRAM: (ailments-conditions)

STRESS (Trigger)
"fight or flight"
nervous system- hyper-excitability

HYPOTHYROIDISM
decreased metabolism: wt. Gain
Hormone Imbalance
irritability
tired

AMYGDALA
"fight or flight"

ADRENAL BURNOUT
increased Cortisol
increased estrogen (decreased testosterone)

MAGNESIUM DEFICIENCY
Increased Ca in soft tissues
Pain, fatigue (decreased energy)
sensitivities: allergies

ANEMIA
decreased iron
decreased energy

SADS: decreased Vit D absorption
insomnia
anxiety
seizures: depression
osteoporosis
diabetes

INFLAMMATION
pain, stiffness, fatigue etc

GLUTEN SENSITIVE
aches; fatigue, insomnia, seizures,
irritability, foggy brain decreased Mg absorption
gut problems= decreased absorption of nutrients
insulin problems/diabetes
increased belly fat: Wt. Gain (more Estrogen; Estrones)
hyperglycemic

Take:

"Mg+"

WITH MAGNESIUM SUPPLEMENTATION: (required)

relief of cramps: relaxation of muscles: no more pain

Energy metabolism: functioning mitochondria (no more fatigue)
decreased blood pressure; **increased cardiovascular function**

calm mind (no more anxiety)
increased bone density
decreased adrenalin/ cortisol: decreased fight or flight

youthfulness; soft skin, no wrinkles
sleep better

rids migraines

no more pain: intercepts pain receptors
opens arteries and veins so better blood flow

decreases inflammation

better nerve transmission
no more foggy brain- clear thinking
less memory problems

wt. loss- due to increased energy and activity

calms amygdala (fight/flight)

helps Depression (so do probiotics help)

HOW FIBRO CREPT BACK INTO MY LIFE

So here we are in January 2015 and I realize I let Fibro back into my life. How did this happen?.....well I had gone off gluten about 90% free for about 18 months and then slowly started back at gluten over the past year or so, getting so bad I'd have a bagel/ day again. Oh no. I felt very tired and lately some body aches and pains so I knew, it was coming to revisit because I fell into bad habits again. Gluten is so easy to let back into your life, you just do a little , then more, then more, then wow you are back to it being 90% of your diet and you feel lousy again. I have brain fog all over again too. How I wish to feel good again, so in being inspired to release my book and get it onto other peoples shelves rather than just my own, I perused it to see the secrets once again. Ah ha, that is what I do. I had forgotten some of it, so it will be handy for you to keep it on the shelf and in your life in case you do what I did, slip back into gluten and old habits.

So yesterday I felt so much like eating a pizza, I did not however, instead I have gone cold turkey with gluten once again to heal my gut, went to the grocery store and bought organic fruits, yogurt, organic beef and gluten free (brown rice) tortillas with some cheese, organic tomatoes and organic turkey to make quesadillas for lunch. The cravings are there but I resist them and remember how ill gluten made me feel and how wonderful I can feel again, enough of this slow self sabotage. Nowadays, there are so many more gluten products then even 3 years ago, so easy to avoid gluten now. I also bought eggs, I believe they are very good for you and they tie over my appetite for hours where I don't feel hungry til noon or early afternoon, (I have eggs for breakfast) then I make a quesadilla for lunch and then have the odd steak for dinner with nibbling on fruits during the day, quinoa and yogurt as snacks too. My fridge is colourful again. Costs a bit more but very worth it and you have to shop smart. I still have my green smoothie in the mornings as I don't find I have enough veggies in my diet, this you have to watch for powders that they don't contain any gluten or you will be frequenting gluten again.

So it should take about 3- 6 months til my gut is a lot better and I can absorb important nutrients and get my energy back. I have not purchased more Mg just yet for pain but just finished some recently, I try to take a maintenance level of 1-2 capsules per day though.

I hope you are more aware and cautious then I, in falling back into the gluten and pain cycle. This is why I include it here, as a forewarning so you don't travel the same path and you can maintain your healthy habits. Being tired, especially in your mid 40's is a real drag, at times I feel like an 80 year old. Discouraging in life. We all wish to feel vitality, and energy gives us this.

So watch your diet at all times and catch yourself if you slip back into eating bagels and feel dragged down or get brain fog back. As soon as you do catch yourself, change your habits back into healthy ones and cut it out cold turkey til you feel better again. Hope this bit of advice and warning helps you. I just went along and thought when I had really felt better …."oh I can do a little gluten again, it won't hurt"….well over time it will do it's damage and you will feel back to square one again.

So keep this book handy as a go to if need be, share with others but always try to get it back and keep it as future reference as it is very applicable and some stuff easy to forget. I personally like reading over the bits I included at the end, easy reads and reminders about life and our struggles.

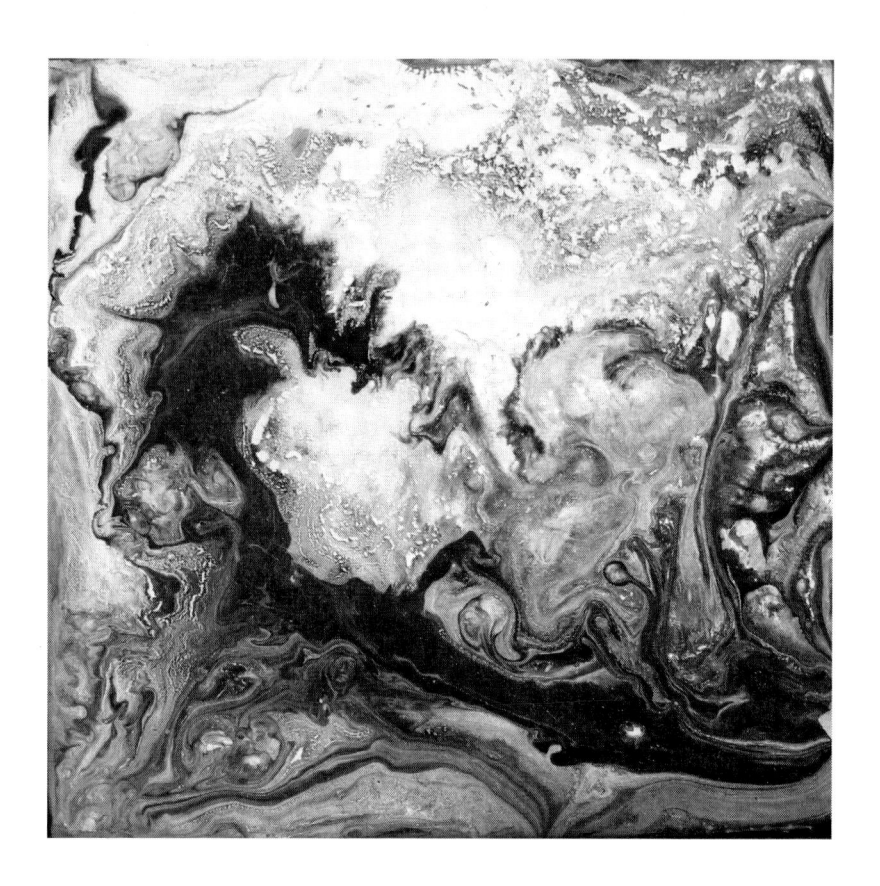

XI. Who is right, the MD or Naturopath?
(Western Medicine vs. Eastern Medicine)

So after all your reading and new found knowledge you ask well who is right, my medical doctor or specialist or is the naturopathic doctor the one who is smarter?

Neither I say, both are required, any one taken to an extreme is incorrect I feel. It is like a happy marriage, they balance each other out if taken together.

You see we need the western stuff like some (only some, lets not over do it like we have!) medicine (drugs) are very helpful and beneficial to many people saving many, many lives. More of a cut and sew approach and put a bandaid on it for now til we truly know how to resolve (and things take time to resolve). Western medicine is very helpful when it comes to emergencies or trauma.

I was saved for instance by a heart surgeon who sewed up a dangerous hole in my heart (ASD) which was life threatening, Eastern medicine would not have been of any help. I was extremely tired etc and instead of taking herbs, which I tried, one day (after 4 years of searching), a doctor said well if you are tired could be your heart, let's take a picture of it and see, so an echo was performed in due course and pow there it was, a big hole in my heart, things got quite serious then. So I was given one year to live if not fixed. I took the surgery obviously thus why I sit here right now penning this book (yes penning). But then on the flip side of things I had this fibromyalgia which no doctor I ever spoke with even believed in it, they would always say it is just in your head, they had no clue, no X-rays or pictures of it. So not really an emergency til it causes a heart attack....til then you slowly suffer in pain, agony and fatigue. Well this is where Eastern medicine comes in is with a Naturopath who looks more internally and subjective and esp your diet, what are you putting in your mouth to cause it? What do you need to do to resolve the underlying issue? Not an emergency or trauma but rather long term suffering which is by far worse. So I discovered what I discuss in this book, missing minerals and gluten preventing Mg from being absorbed, what little we now get from food, a vitamin/mineral deficiency which modern western medical doctors still don't relate to or are not taught about unless they self learn.

One cannot be narrow minded, even in life, one has to be open to "new" ideas or thoughts whether a new drug or new disease. And real solutions look at what is the cause not effect. So there you have it Eastern looks at cause and Western deals with the effect (depends where we are on the spectrum which help we need). I firmly believe in both and in alot of ways have become my own doctor, knowing firstly myself and luckily having a science base (pre-med degree) and the internet and friends who help me with the rest. I put it all together according to how it helps and works for myself and get good results. I am now so healthy and only getting better. I am thankful for both (all) practices of health and illness.

Who can really say who is right, it is all an individual game, we all have individual bodies just as we have individual personalities, western generalizes and averages us , eastern treats us as unique individuals. I really like we have both ! **It is all about balance.**

XII. CONCLUSION:

Fibro is such a mystery to most, what I present is tried and true for myself after alot of other methods and struggles, it is thru my hard work and time and paying attention to what works and finding out why and how, that I have come to write this book. I might be way off but I may be RIGHT ON, you be the judge, it takes minimal time, effort and cash to try my methods and my only hope is to help just one person, so maybe that is you? Maybe after reading this book and trying, and if it works, you can pass the book onto your family doctor and help educate them with this worthy point of view of fibromyalgia, the mystery alot of people don't believe in. Well I know it exists and while you will always have those small few who take advantage and maybe fake it to get something, alot of people genuinely suffer and must be helped to have a healthier life and fulfilment and be out of pain. I believe I have just 'connected all the dots' here and I really hope people will find it beneficial in their lives, it took me over 2 years to write and I did it in longhand first, so alot of work but a nice journey and good process I have enjoyed. I love to help others if I am truly able and they want to truly help themselves.

I feel it is a combination of contributing factors and all must be resolved:
1. Mg deficient
2. Gluten/ inflammation
3. The Amygdala
4. Ca in tissues due to low Mg
5. Adrenal burnout/ thyroid issues
6. stress/trauma

My book covers all these.

Follow my simple steps and hopefully you too will regain your life and footing and also contribute. Above all, Be PATIENT and try to figure out what works for you individually as we are all individuals, alot of problems do exist I believe because of poor diets though.
Unfortunately we live in such a 'convenient' world in this day that we don't take time for proper nutrition (nor do some farmers) on which our bodies are based, along with our thoughts. Remember thoughts are powerful, they feed us too and mold who we are and who we become. Get rid of old patterns or bad habits, form new healthy ones, only you can truly help yourself. Start today!

"Precisely WHAT we think today, tomorrow will bring"
(jemma)

"You can change, start today"

"Patience is always rewarded"

"Our thoughts bring reality"   (jemma)

"You cannot pursue your passion(s) when there is conflict"

"Our greatest fears can become reality when we give them life, breath" (jemma)

"Priorities, choices, whatever time we put into or spend on something is not going into putting it in another" (jemma)

"You can't be angry and thankful at the same time"

"The lows in life make us appreciate the good times even more"

"Some things we read about and some we live, mostly you have to live it to really know it " (Jemma)

"Usually what people say of others is true about themselves"

"Our age is not a gauge of our wisdom......just our experience"

"The higher you climb or feel, the longer and harder the ride down, stay in the middle" (jemma)

"Don't engage in negative emotions or negative talk"

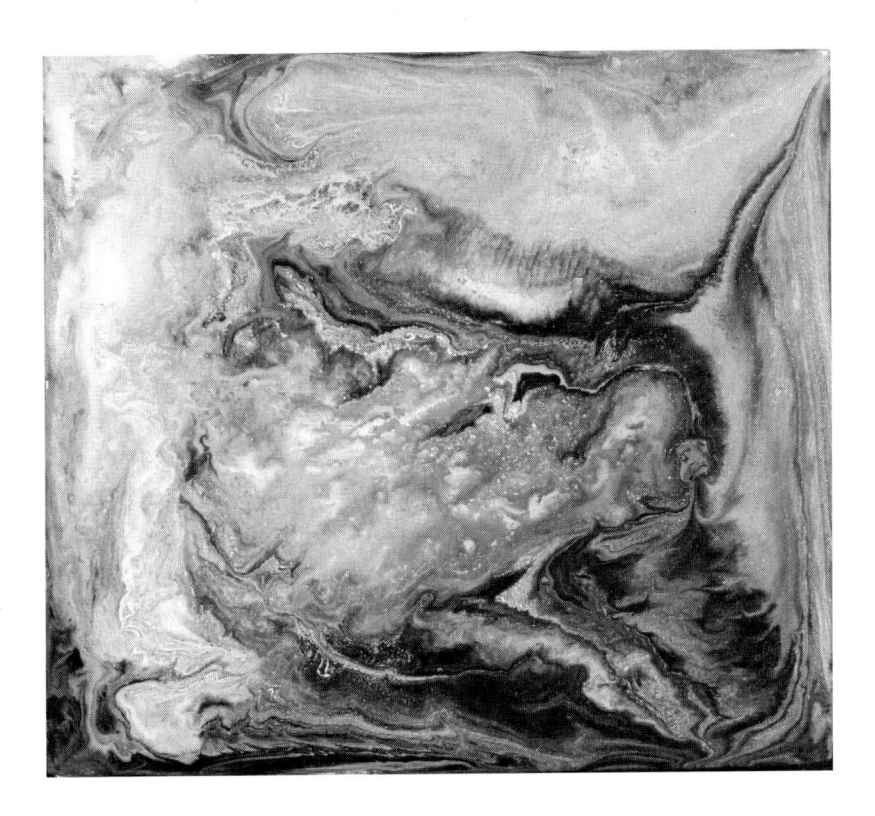

PART 4

DEPRESSION - IN MORE DETAIL

Depression what is it, how does it happen and how can we help it.

I will just cover the basics here as there are many great books on depression and thus will not go into alot of detail.

Probiotics and the Brain:

IMPORTANT: The newest research out now is how probiotics (good gut bacteria) impact people with depression, mental illness even, it helps them, this makes complete sense because a healthy gut does often determine a healthy mind, they are deeply connected. The gut produces around 70-90% of the serotonin in the body the brain uses and without a healthy gut producing this, you may fall into some depression in life. But good news and this is groundbreaking, by getting a healthy gut again and putting probiotics into it to help the healthy bacteria flourish you can help regain your brain! I won't say much more here about it except you can google the topic and learn about all the new research yourself, just find the right probiotic for you and try to take when needed or regularly especially after taking high doses of antibiotics as this wipes out your good and bad bacteria together. If the bad bacteria out populates the good , you are sure to have gut problems and digestion issues. (and feel blue) They have also found recently that there is a huge nerve connecting the gut to the brain, this leading to that old adage when something doesn't feel right, "it is just a gut feeling". That is your mind communicating with your gut. (maybe a form of intuition ?).

Depression:

Depression is where the person doesn't feel well (down) mainly in the head but it does affect the body too. Nobody really knows how it begins except that there is a genetic factor involved which may increase one's vulnerability when combined with environment and personality. Mainly women outnumber men in statistically coming down with depression. I believe this is because of hormones mainly and how they play a role in structuring the brain as well as it has to do with the level of sensitivity and emotional response. Definitely men are more successful when it comes to suicide, there is more of a finality to it. Whereas women will not be as successful and are more likely to seek therapy and talk it out. Men are very good at hiding it thus partly the reason for the lower statistic as well(?).

There's also a connection to trauma and loss, Financial difficulties (strife), as well as one's personality such as being a perfectionist. Stress is a big factor in triggering depression I believe. The better one manages stressors in their life, the less prone they're likely to

come down with depression. There are vitamins and medications which assist with depression which I will go into later the main ones being vitamin B's, omega-3's and vitamin D. For the brain one really needs healthy oils and B12 as well as folic acid. The brain is full of nerves and one is constantly regenerating these nerves (I believe) and thus we need to assist this process by good nutrition. Depression is very much a mind, body, Spirit ailment as it involves emotions, thought, behaviour and physiology.
Most people who don't have depression don't understand it and just see the outward behaviour of people who suffer and as a result are very often hard on them emotionally and physically, this all leading to great difficulty in relationships for the people who suffer depression. It is imperative Family members and spouses relate to and understand how this person suffers and what they're dealing with and that if it isn't dealt with, that possible outcomes end in tragedy. Depression has many levels and severity and will fluctuate between feeling okay one-day to feeling really bad another.

When one suffers depression you're highly unmotivated, Withdraw from activities/society, have difficulty getting chores done as well as the to do list which grows up like a mountain, you are easily overwhelmed, Have difficulty concentrating and often, if not always, have an accompanying sleep disorder. Fatigue can kick in and be a result of depression. This fatigue which can be debilitating, as one can become fixated on it. It is important to maintain A regular sleep schedule, Quality sleep, as well as taking naps during the day as required. Most often an ear mark of depression is getting up early say 4 a.m. If one feels fresh enough to get up at this hour you should utilize your time either get a couple chores done, Clean a bit, Take care of yourself and self-care, Journal or do hobbies. The best time I find I function is between 4 AM and 8 AM, this is the time I tend to write, I can think best and am most motivated (it is also very quiet). My energy is the most high at this time. The rest of the day I use to do a couple chores, Indulge in activities that I enjoy whether just going for a walk and cup of coffee or watching a favourite TV show and spend some time meditating as well as catching up on e-mails and business like opening mail and responding.

I must now implement exercise regularly into my regime too as it is vital to good health and conquering depression. I still have too many bad days I wish to resolve esp as of late and I believe thru exercise it will help. It is important one doesn't overdo it one day and "fall down" and then have things pile up into the following week as this can seem very overwhelming and builds into a mountain (added stress). One must take baby steps and do a little at a time and think positive whenever possible as people with depression tend to think more negative and focus on the negative versus the positive, hope and optimism. But we can help control our brains by catching these negative thoughts and turning them around as soon as possible and possibly this'll have an effect on what is called 'neuro-plasticity' which is forming new nerve associations in the brain and perhaps negative thoughts are black and positive thoughts are white and we could think of it as trying to produce more white and take out the black. Nobody knows how these connections are made except the negative thoughts are more powerful and have more connections (shown on MRI's) and for us are more memorable than pleasurable moments or positive things. There's so much unknown about the mind, So much to be discovered.

It is recently noted that it is actually not a "biochemical imbalance" that occurs with depression, that this theory has been created by marketing teams of pharmaceutical companies trying to sell drugs which they insist try to correct this biochemical imbalance thus their solution and how they make money. The role of serotonin on depression is still up in the air and nobody really knows its effect. People through practice just know what seems to work for depressed patients and help heal them so they may come out of it. A lot of this practice is around psychotherapy, talk therapy, some medication and a dose of exercise.

One cannot seclude themselves and become isolated for this makes it worse, (you dwell more), one must try to engage in minor activities working their way up to the regular activities they used to enjoy, one step at a time and with discipline. This forms new pleasurable connections in the brain, the healthy ones which spur you on towards greater health and wellbeing (create good, positive habits, one at a time). It will give you a lift and sense of accomplishment when you tackle and complete little tasks, one at a time. This in turn will build confidence and much needed self esteem, keeping one on the positive road to recovery.

It's been proven by research that exercise is as beneficial if not more than medication or even medication combined with exercise. When one exercises the chance of 'relapse' is a lot less. It is been stated by professionals that Depression and it's problem far Outweighs that of Heart Disease. This is especially seen in North America. My theory is that it is tied into our lack of exercise plus lack of nutrition and higher stress levels in this first world (associated with our now lack of proper and solid communication and concrete social networks falling apart). So much of our world relates to money now and with money it carries stress whether on a subconscious level or conscious. People recognize money as security and feel safe when they have more of it. People always want to feel safe and not fearful. In the state of becoming safe often people become selfish and narcissistic (we all want to win the lottery nowadays). These features are also an aspect of the North American Society which exists. Money is essentially just numbers on paper that go up and come down, just like stocks. Sure it is good and healthy to have some money to care for one self and their family but know how much you need and what will suffice without stressing you or stretching you beyond your means, live below your means and stay away from credit as it is a real stressor and very unrealistic to pay later (you pay a lot more), banks and drug companies rule too much over North American society and have become uncompassionate giants.

A lot of North America focuses still on Western medicine too and is controlled greatly by the pharmaceutical companies who have one focus and that is mainly profits. North America needs more Eastern influence, more communication, Empathy and compassion involved in it's medical approach. Depression should not be such a big problem but I agree it is on the rise and we must take a strong look at it and try to resolve it believing in prevention versus a cure. People with depression are not weak in character, rather I feel they are just a little more sensitive and prone to stress whether due to genetics or environment and if all factors combine it will trigger this illness of depression which is hard to undo once initiated.

So with this lack of motivation, negative thinking and fatigue it is very hard to build a life and feel good about yourself. So many people including yourself see yourself as a failure when in actuality you are just going through a time of reflection, Healing and merely a phase. Is important one sees that it is a phase and that one can get better (that it is temporary). Hope, optimism and positive thinking and heading in the right direction, if one does not want a boring life, is Key to recovery. There's also an affliction called bipolar which I will not go into for it is out of context within this book. It is also very complicated to discuss and recover from if one ever recovers. We could look at depression as being the light form of bipolar and thus possibly more resolvable. One often has difficulties controlling cycles when bipolar vs. just a constant down mood with depression. A roller coaster is much more difficult to contain and deal with in life. Tho many will attest to the benefits of the highs. (highly motivated and dreamer, risk taker)

So how does one resolve depression you ask. Great question. As covered, exercise is very important, Nutrition is key, and controlling and managing your thoughts is imperative as well. Just catch yourself and use discipline in all these departments. Insight and reflection are great tools for recovery. Journaling can be very helpful to see progress and how far you've come and also releasing anxiety and stress which assists in healing. Exercise can be any form of fast walking to running, Yoga, swimming or team sport where you are active. It is important you get the heart rate up, to circulate the blood and in a sense cleanse the brain of toxins and stress and I believe very much that exercise has a strong impact on healthy sleeping and will help resolve sleep disorders which are deeply tied into depression. Experts are unclear of how exercise helps just that it does, thru research it has been proven. I just tend to believe that circulating the blood throughout the body is cleansing and gets everything where it needs to be while removing anything that is a detriment physically to the body and this is akin to fresh oil running in your car. Circulating the blood cleans out all the garbage and gets much-needed oxygen, especially to the brain. For it is oxygen, water and nutrients that run our body.

Within the brain we have thoughts, some people feel first, some people think first, but they're tied together and we must try to control our anger which can result from negative thinking. When you think a negative thought or catch yourself, quickly stop it in your mind especially if it runs as a movie and replace it with the other side of the coin which will be positive. Always try to see the positive in people and situations (outcomes), that will make you a lot happier in life and more stress-free. We always find what we look for whether the positive or negative. Negative for some reason effects our body detrimentally and makes it unhealthy whereas positive has a different "frequency"(as discussed earlier) and for some reason this energy assists in healing and makes us healthy. Much like a good nutrient or vitamin or sound. Nobody has ever failed or been hurt by thinking positively.

So in conclusion, one must exercise, sometimes take medication, control their sleep patterns and/or thought patterns and try their best at relationships, not isolate themselves unless they are naturally a recluse (which most aren't - we are naturally social animals), get out and do activities or do hobbies which Elevate the spirit and in doing so, this increases the Good neurotransmitters in the brain and helps assist neuro-plasticity. One must definitely find a way to decrease their stress whether 'getting things done' or 'tackling any thinking patterns', have a release such as yoga or exercise or journaling or meditation. It is imperative one controls their stress in order to recover from depression. I myself don't exercise enough but like to walk, I will start rigorously exercising as I feel blue lately, my nutrition is pretty good and my thought patterns are well-managed. I have a tremendous amount of stress in my life which I manage and most people would buckle under but I hold such a good positive attitude towards a good outcome that it tends not to stress me out. I try to take one step at a time and not jumping into the future or live in the past. Relationships are certainly an area one must work on and every day try to improve. I try to remain trustworthy and flexible with others with a good dose of compassion. I realize that everybody has their life, their own problems and don't really want to share in yours, they just want to hear the positive and not get dragged down by the negative. This I can respect as for what we used to call friends are now called paid psychologists, just an unfortunate reality of living in 2014. It is only with people I truly trust– I share my problems with and use as a sounding board but only in small doses, without overwhelming them, when you are too intense or problematic, are always one way and then another, people get frustrated and will remove themselves from your life and you will find yourself even more isolated.

You must become more gentle with yourself and others and be your own best friend and feed yourself complements all the time as you cannot expect to hear it from others (love yourself unconditionally). People are just too busy to complement others nowadays. It seems we'd rather focus on the negative than the positive, just a human aspect and how our brains operate. We must learn to love unconditionally, to help each other, as for this is very rewarding and heals the soul and feeds the spirit and eventually in doing this will heal the body. It never hurts to help somebody out or at least try. For that is the reason I believe we are all here and find our journey and purpose, is in using our specific skills and talents to assist others out of their pain or where they are weak and make this a better journey, one of evolving rather than destruction.

It is very important to communicate above all when one is depressed, Reach out for help as there are a lot of people out there who understand and know how to help you. Never be afraid to ask for help as you're stronger in doing so rather than seeing yourself as weak. There is great strength in revealing vulnerability. We all have our times we need help and we need people to lean on. You should feel confident and strong and be open to discuss with those you trust how you are feeling, what you're going through and ask how you can get help.

I hope some of these insights help you as I hope some of your own insights help you. I do wish more people would seek help rather than the alternative of ending their lives without seeing their purpose to fruition while on earth. It is sad for all, mostly those left behind as they always feel woulda, shoulda, coulda and there's always regret and guilt, two very hard things to live with and recover from.

By discussion and communication and openness, we can help a lot of people survive this illness, Overcome it and conquer it. If ever you feel you having a bad day, just go to bed early, wake up the next day and it'll be a new opportunity to feel differently, usually I do this and this works for me, Always.

So never see it is the end, don't feel you are alone and don't feel there's no one out there to help you because there is and yes you will get better.

One important mood stabilizer I find in my life (as a women esp) that works is Evening Primrose Oil, helps balance hormones and tame an angry personality or spirit, you can be more yourself rather than your hormones. I much prefer this over say lithium to control mood. Never have tried lithium mind you.

Always get your blood work done too as hypothyroidism (as I discuss in this book) can easily disguise as depression, along with other illnesses or diseases. You must know the beast you are dealing with in order to conquer it!

Randy Peterson….has a clinic called 'Change Ways' on broadway in Vancouver BC, he said alot in a talk one night, some of which I try to repeat here for assistance:

About depression: is that you should set your goals for everyday living lower and achieve small steps and that exercise helps a lot. You should also engage in activities and with others to get out of funks, all this I agree with. Good advice. Randy said instead of just trying harder, give up, throw in the towel and set your expectations low, I believe this then feeds into your self esteem and positive thinking patterns and gives one a "lift" in life. Randy also has a book out (focus is depression).

When you think about it we are all creatures of habit and just like we fell into depression, we can fall back out of it. Create positive and healthy habits, daily and religiously and build and create the life you wish to have and enjoy and who you' like to enjoy it with, always see the positive and above all, " always be thankful". For instance, start your morning, like oh thank god I am still alive and have a beautiful useful day ahead of me where I may help serve others. Be thankful for simply breathing, life will get a lot simpler.
Don't build mountains out of molehills, see everything for the size it really is and how valuable it is or isn't to you. See my writings on 'life is a canvas' where I talk about building a painting of your life. Once we create enough healthy thoughts and habits and come to appreciate more the little things again we will soon as if by magic walk into the life we desire. As like overnight successes, it may take many years to create this. Keep steady and keep working

towards it, build it like you would a business you would want to work in. Make it rewarding and fruitful and build emotional security rather than money based security which can easily fall apart. Soon it will serve you instead of you it. Enjoy life above all and persevere, as it is getting thru the tough times where we really evolve and can serve and find purpose and meaning which is what we all ultimately seek, whether subconsciously or consciously. Try not to use people either but rather a give and take and paying it forward attitude, this will serve you better as people will always figure out if you are a manipulator or user and not appreciate the abuse of it. Give and take remember that, balance. And never be afraid you are " being used" either, take it in stride as you are just helping, for one day they will wake and see your value.

Most of all, speak out, ask for help as help always exists.

note : Be careful, sometimes medications side effects can often be depression.

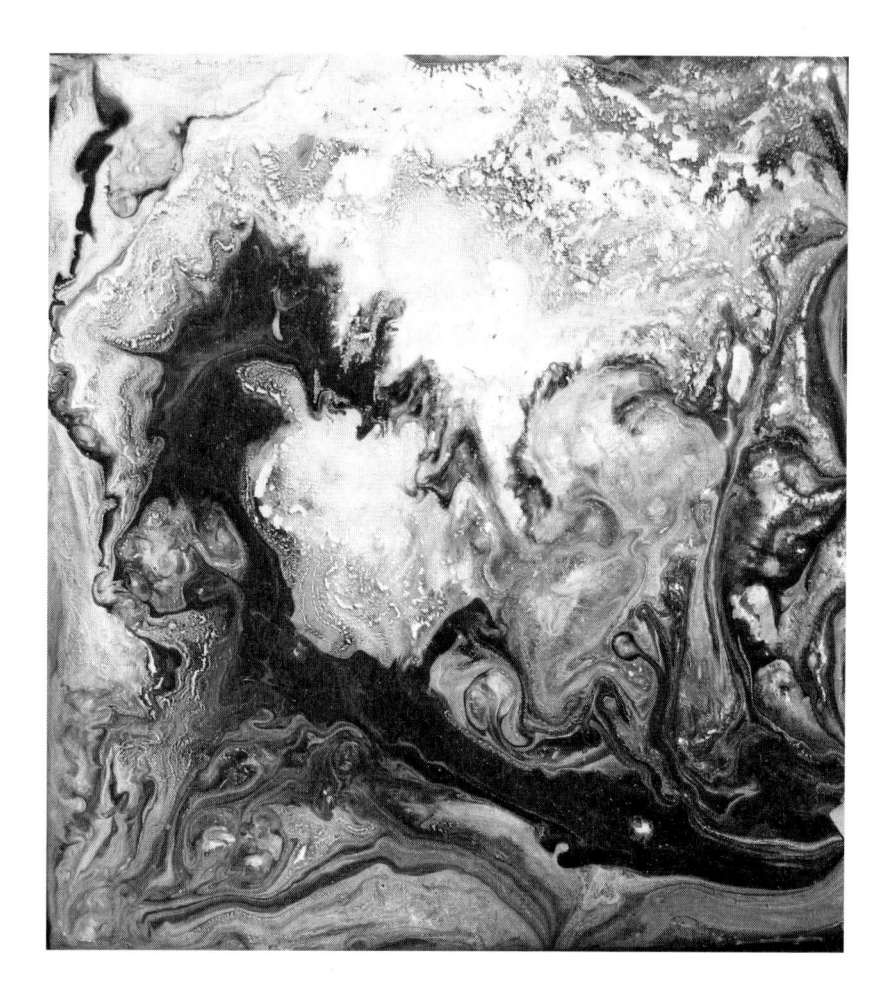

PART 5 :

XIII RANDOM RELATED TOPICS

Why I Wrote This Book:

I have survived many things in my life and recovered successfully, fibro being just one of them. Sure I could have kept my success and secrets and knowledge, experience to myself but I thought why not write it down and make a book, it can't be too hard and although writing is not my forte, I saw it as a healthy challenge.

My intent is I thought if I could help "one" person recover and be better that would make it all worth my efforts. For I know how much it means to me to beat fibro and have my health back and if I could do that for one or for many, that would be a great thing and make it meaningful that I happened to get fibro and did figure alot of it out. I have thus turned "Pain into Purpose", the best way to deal with it. I am also one to want to help others. I feel I have learned great compassion and patience and understanding. I was not like this in my 20's but rather gained it thru my life experiences. It would be a waste if me, having all this time, did nothing to try to help others, to not contribute. I cannot imagine how I would feel, as well as others if this book actually holds alot of truths and they be studied and actually work for a wide range of people. I would be elated to learn that this book is truly cutting edge info and helps doctors better understand the illness so they may help. I have not read any book of this sort out there or seen one so I feel it is unique and again just a true story of my individual journey of suffering and success.

Fibro seems to be so mysterious to many but not to me. It has taken me several years to piece it together, mostly alot done this past 8 months or so and people I find have mixed reviews on me writing it. Which I don't care. People seem to either react when I tell them about me writing this book like
a. they don't care
b. they question it and think impossible (cure)
c. they get jealous and react in jest or negatively
d. some are very supportive and interested.
Mostly c. So I told very few if any people and only some during the last stages of finishing it off as the excitement in me grew of sharing my story and success and hoping that for others as well. I've learned you have to pick and choose who you tell big ideas or dreams to , as they can immediately judge and this then impacts your journey or path you are on. So be selective in sharing your dreams; tell only those who will support you and be positive for and with you. For I believe anything is possible when you put

effort and time and work into it. Everyone has a story to tell, not all successes but that's ok too as we can still all learn.

Did I really have fibro you may wonder, YES, I truly had fibro, as I had CFS in my early 20's for years/decades with mono @ 18-19 and been thru trauma and long term stress (leading to adrenal burnout) and I had all the pressure points, pain and all symptoms, nearly used a cane to walk and really had almost worse than anyone else I knew. I know exactly what you are going thru, have been thru and hold hope you too can get all better. It is with utter excitement I share my findings and story with you as I feel we gain much when we communicate and share- someone will listen, pay attention and benefit.

"Luck is on your side, you just have to work for it." (jemma)

CHANGE:

Yes, change is hard but usually it's for the better. We can get so "stuck" and comfortable even if in a painful spot or difficult situation for us. Even so when we are in a good spot and stuck it is also hard to move even more forward in life and accept change. Right now I am going thru change and personally I feel scared. Scared because it feels so big, unknown and will be so different for me but such a big move in my life forward and to a happier place. I feel comfortable with the pain and challenges I am presently experiencing- it feels familiar and almost "normal" to me. Change feels like such unknown territory and as humans we like to know where we are going, how long it will take and when we will be there. (much like driving). The unexpected or out of the norm can feel awkward and induce fear. But, one must step up to this fear and face it in the eyes and say to oneself, I welcome change, bring it on, I deserve better than where I am presently at.

It takes steps, one at a time to reach a goal where there is such change. Work everyday towards this goal and sooner or later you will be at your goal and it will feel like it was so easy.
"Why all the fear"? you will take a breath and say. You'll say to yourself: This is so much better than before, I must just adjust to this new environment, respect, job, habits, etc.

We can often feel like we don't deserve better, either self-esteem issues (which we all have), insecurities or self destructive thinking issues. This we must get beyond, day by day working towards self preservation, health, respect for oneself and getting it from others (as a result of having it for yourself) and fight for what we feel is right, just and good for ourselves. Either psychotherapy works for bettering self- esteem, or simply exercising or meditation work just as well too I find. I practice meditation myself, a time where I "feed" my mind a healthy diet of good thoughts, aspirations, dreams, self-reflection and positive energy. Meditation is something you give yourself for yourself, like a gift. I meditate every am and before sleep. With enough time of disciplined practice, just like a sore muscle healing and getting rehab, you will one day just find yourself there- thinking
"I do deserve better and I 'm going after it!"
Speaking from personal experience it is alot easier to adjust to 'good' and people treating you well than treating you badly. Hurt is not healthy. **So realize your self worth and live it.**

"In losing something (ie. job, someone), we are given the opportunity to find something even better"

"Everyone is lucky,......few are prepared".

"It's darkest before the light"

"Is the fear of change greater than the pain you are suffering"?

FIBROSUCCESS

SEXUAL ABUSE/ PHYSICAL ABUSE

There is a strong connection between fibro and past sexual or physical abuse or a traumatic event. This I believe falls into place in the scenario of fibro as when you are abused as a child or even as an adult it shows itself in insidious stress. This stress takes a toll on the adrenals, eventually burning them out. A traumatic event or injury can have the same effect except more of a larger hit over less time period but still same result. Just the fact of having fibro burns the adrenals out further also, as you are under alot of stress and duress being ill.

Sexual abuse is very much a touchy subject. I have a friend (we'll call her Sam), she was sexually abused throughout life by her father. I don't truly and deeply understand the issue wholly as I have not experienced it myself. But I do understand a bit about it and abuse itself whether sexual, mental, emotional or physical. My friend Sam told me recently she was calling her dad to touch base, I replied that is odd, what about all the sexual abuse, have you forgiven him and want a relationship? She said to me "well being in the field I am in (mental therapist) I obviously understand why people do the things they do , so....." I thought hhhhmmm, she said it was a "courtesy call" back to him and that when he dies she doesn't want any regrets. Odd I thought. He seems to be in complete denial about it and not accept responsibility, this must be so hard on her to be in contact with him and have any sort of connection. (she is going thru alot of pain right now, mental and physical). With abusers, just because you understand why they do/did what they do doesn't mean you have to "accept it" and be a part of their life. Unless both parties are very clear on the past and what happened and dealt with it, I do not see how it could be a healthy relationship between abusee and abuser. I feel it is super she is forgiving as we all have to be, as if we're not, it hurts only us and continues memories of abuse and hurts. So forgive and let go but don't feel obligated to accept this person back into your life if not healthy for you, blood or not.

You will feel no regret at the end of the day being at peace with them and the situ. If they die in denial or without you that is all about them, not you.

Even if people seem to have valid reasons or excuses for doing such heinous things to others esp family, they need to first recognize they did it and then take responsibility and hopefully apologize and ask forgiveness. If they don't do this and they remain a part of your life, a part of you remains in denial of what you went thru. Feel, Deal and Heal and pick those who are truly healthy for you to be around or recovery is near impossible.

I feel no regrets with my father (who was very abusive) when he passed. I feel free. And although he never took responsibility and we did not have a good relationship, I have no regrets in keeping my distance from his 'poison'. I am sure wherever he is, he is learning and has many regrets, but me no, I was fortunate to say "I love you" as he took his last breath (via phone) and this gave me much needed closure. So you can tell them you love them, etc and be there for them when they are ready to be a healthy part of your life but for the time they remain toxic to you, keep your distance and sanity and always remember that you didn't (never) deserved it, that you are worthy and deserve to heal and let go. Take it as a bad event you recovered from and deal with it on your own individual healthy terms whether alone or with that abuser. Be healthy and worthy of better.

Don't let the fact you were sexually or physically abused define you or your future. Let the scars go, the victim mentality and deal with it and let it all go, all the anger, it's not healthy to hang onto. I know this will be hard, if not impossible. Don't let it hold you back in life from all you "can become" or "have" (ie. A loving mate and /or success) Don't let the fact it happened (and yes it's hard) DICTATE in life why you "can't" or "not have". Don't let it become an "excuse". Go for all you deserve in life with the new found compassion and insight the abuse gave you, use it to help others recover and move on . Tame the beast it is and release it. Feel , deal and heal and let it go (give it closure once and for all).

Get it OUT of your life so it can no longer harm you. Forgive and move on (forward).

"Love and Care for what you Have, not want".

HOW WE FEEL ABOUT OTHERS IN OUR LIFE (HAVING A MATE)

Several women I've talked to with Fibro state to me that they are alone because of Fibro and that they can barely look after themselves and don't wish to involve another into their situ. This is very true for many. Whether Fibro helped dissolve a marriage for women in particular or whether they have just remained single due to not getting out and being able to put on a good front. It is hard to get to know new people and date when you have fibro- there are alot of inconsistent days and not too many people understand when you share the info you have it. They tend to think oh oh do I want to deal with this too?

As women are seen as the care provider in relationships with men I tend to believe that often men, when sick with fibro, are better cared for and relationships remain intact as the women in their life helps care for them and get their health back. True, men are mainly the bread winner and this puts a strain on things but women generally have a stick by your side attitude. So when a women gets fibro I can see how men would generally give up and leave as they would often feel neglected and their compassion (only sometimes) is lower than a women, at times. Not saying all though. Men are very good care providers just that in North America a women's role still remains largely the caregiver and housewife (even tho we have made great strides). So when a man falls ill the women may often get work to support the family while the man remains sick and tired at home. This way a women does double duty (work and caregiver).
It takes a very strong person to stand by someone with fibro and it

often is akin to one with MS-not really seen but very difficult and painful to deal with. At first glance one wants to question their partner (I went thru this with my heart situ and fiance). Questioning is not healthy when all one needs is support. Support and answers and resolutions. Communication is key to any relationship and especially I find when one party is suffering so. You do say in sickness and in health after all, good times and bad, unfortunately some don't stick to this.

How it Creeps Up on You:

So CFS or fibro are of a slow progression, sometimes though can be immediate. If one suffers an acute trauma, they can fall ill within several months afterwards. However for most under long term stress the body slowly takes a hit. It comes on so slowly til one day you can't get out of bed and your body just aches all over. How did this come about you wonder ? slowly. I believe the adrenals burnout due to stress, the Amygdala is kicked into high gear. Plus Ca is in the tissues causing contraction due to fight or flight response to adrenalin and cortisol. The buildup towards full blown fibro takes time and is rather a slow progression. It feels then when you are finally diagnosed after seeing several doctors and /or specialists, it feels too late to do something substantial to rid you of it. Basically, it will take a toll on your body and start destroying one organ at a time with all the inflammation. Genetics will often determine the weakest, most prone organ to disease and that may go first. You feel like you are dying and slowly and painfully your systems are breaking down and being destroyed (taxed) so in reality this is what is happening. But there is plenty of hope, once one is diagnosed they try to manage this fibro and some are quite successful. Management feels so slow and one must always take proper steps and pace oneself. It feels too slow, we all want to be better tomorrow! Well with this book I hope you can get beyond just management and be cured, live a full and happy life again. I believe it's possible and within 3-6 months I felt like a brand new person. I tend to believe tho it takes approx.

1 year to be alot better as your organs (esp gut) need time and care to repair, but they can and will. The body is an amazing strong and smart machine (tool). The brain will come back, stress will go down, rest will improve (which is key to repairing) and exercise will re-enter your life. Work on the body, mind and spirit all simultaneously not as separate and your recovery will progress speedingly quicker. Listen to your body and what works and what you need- keep a "food and feel" journal (what you eat and how it makes you feel), this will be a good tool.

Continue with the things that seem to work and drop those things that don't. Try to analyze your individuality and individual situ with fibro as we are all different and the range of fibro is a big scale from mild to severe for some. Take steps every day toward better health and sooner or later one day you will wake up and find you are there- healthy again and willing to create new important relationships. You will learn that you can be more consistent with "showing up" and you will learn to depend on yourself and your health more, as so will others. People will come around and support you as they witness your hard work.

Hopefully the support you need will be there from beginning to end. You will find that special someone in your life and I believe they will be true as they will be supportive and loving. Just be brave and open to finding them- they are out there. I believe there is someone for everyone.
You can and will get better- believe this strongly. Believing is the first step to success!

VULNERABILITY, REJECTION AND BULLYING

To be vulnerable is to be brave. Too many people hide behind a veil, are not real or put on a front. We have gotten to the point where we call this 'being professional" (which can be important).Yes there is being professional but we have gotten to the point where people are so fake and their behaviour so controlled we now expect it from all (and a certain level). It seems people try very hard to control how others behave or act. We don't have this control, it is an illusion and only causes frustration and stigma. It is the ego that likes this control. People who cannot control others being a certain way as expected by the other causes the person to have and feed into stigma. We have to learn to allow people to be themselves and indulge in who they really are, rather than who we think they should be.

Alot of people don't trust people with their vulnerabilities and truths, sometimes their weaknesses. When people show you their true selves you should respect that they trust you enough and thus be gentle and accepting. Our compassion and empathy is at an all time low as our main form of communication is cell phones which we have learned to control, who we want to talk to and when we will talk to them. Cellphones feed the ego and a persons self esteem (even tho not real self esteem). We delete, text, turn off and power on conversations. Technology has ingeniously fed into peoples insecurities and their need to feel power over others. I myself don't have or carry a cell phone, I don't need one. (only some people really do). I have a house phone if someone needs to connect. I don't need a "leash" or a feeling to stay connected where ever I go. I am secure enough to be "alone" and left alone and leave others alone at times. I like not having a cellphone, actually love it. People buy into the fact it adds a layer of security, this being born out of unrealistic fear. Texting is addicting too. The cell phone co.s are smart, they have us by our ears with insecurities and addictions. Big money for them and a loss for you. A loss of money, freedom and privacy. The phones track everywhere you go and apparently can record every conversation. Alot, if not all people, have fallen into this trap.

We are afraid to be vulnerable and real as everything is public and can go viral now. A possibility of embarrassment (widespread). So we hide more. Realness and vulnerability is certainly at an all time low in our society. All people cover up, protect and act. When people are real, it scares us, makes us feel awkward as it has now become so foreign and unacceptable to be real. Relationships suffer as they are superficial and frail with a lack of a real strong support.

People are not real or behave vulnerable because they fear "rejection". Our ego cannot take rejection. Our self esteem is nowadays based on our exterior, what we project and how others perceive us. Money is a root of this.

We do alot for money now. How much money one has is deeply connected to how we feel and it shouldn't be this way. Who we truly are and how we help or treat others should be the core of our self esteem, knowing our talents and abilities and kindness should lead to security and confidence. In our society we focus on how a person dresses for example (ie. a suit) and people dress a certain way because they fear rejection and lack of respect. People admire people who dress well. You know what I admire, someone who works hard, has integrity and treats others, especially the most vulnerable with respect. Earned admiration, not a piece of clothing purchased with money. We all fall into the trap. I try not to. I dress how I feel but when necessary dress for the occasion. I ignore peoples titles for the most part and look at what I admire. Titles sometimes mean nothing if you don't have integrity behind them.

I don't fear rejection, at least I try my best not to. Often if you feel rejected it is more your responsibility how you feel than others. People cannot make you feel small without your permission! I remain myself and real and will wear whatever I feel like dressing in and behave in such a way as I am myself and truly express myself while being what is called professional and respectful towards others. Alot of people cannot handle my realness. They think I am weird or eccentric. Sure, maybe I am a little, but I am not harmful and hurtful towards others and feel their judgement towards me says more about them then it does me. No one can ever get inside your body or mind and know exactly who you are, so don't worry about their perceptions and judgements. I talk alot about this in my section 'people's perceptions of others'.

So be yourself, be BRAVE, real and don't fear rejection. None of us like to feel rejected because it goes against humans wanting to feel connected (a need). The worst of rejection leads to bullying. People bully because they hate themselves, are angry and insecure. They don't feel connected. Some are sociopaths and lack empathy so bullying is in their nature. Bullying hurts, even kills. It is so preventable too. People just need to be called on bullying others and when they treat others with disrespect. This may make the bully mad but better them be put in their place and hear you and be upset then it take a toll on you. Bullying takes a toll on a persons self confidence and self-love. People have inner demons and what bullys have the ability to do is feed these demons or add to them. If too many demons and they are too loud, people will cave to them and eventually end their life to quiet the demons.

Demons can be controlled, they are just negative thoughts or scars and can be replaced with positive, healthy ones. Healing ones. We can quiet the demons but we need to avoid the bully or put them in their place if stuck with them (say co-worker). It must be brought to their attention the affect they have on others, how they hurt and injure others and to stop it. They need help with themselves too. They need to control their bad behaviour. They need lessons in compassion and understanding. If they plainly lack empathy (sociopath) there is no helping them as this is just how their brain is wired. But for most, they will have empathy and when pointed out to them, how they impact and hurt others they will likely stop and change their ways. It takes openness and communication and bravery to stand up to them.

We need to take the power of words more seriously as they can kill, unnecessarily.

At minimum, share your feelings with a confidant and get their opinion on what to do. Maybe they can help you present it to the bully. You are never alone. Some bullys are running rampant now as they feel more powerful with social media. Bullying is far more extreme now then simply a little fight in the back alley of the schoolyard. It is far reaching and more dangerous now. We lose precious lives because these insecure bullies feel a need for power. SAD. We need to take a serious stand and say no more will this disrespectful behaviour be allowed to continue. Bullys should be helped themselves while shunned and rejected for their behaviour. This will squelsh their ego and need for control and power over others. What comes around, goes around and eventually bullies learn their own lessons and can fall victim to it themselves in life.

We all need to learn to treat all humans, no matter position in life, disability or income, with respect. It they are breathing, they deserve love not hate. Bullying is plainly hate. Bullys need to learn love. But above all, realize that you can love yourself in the midst of people hating on you whether rejection or bullying. Be stronger than it. Squelsh it (demons) with all your positive thoughts, tell yourself you are the better person then them and show them love and compassion like yourself. This way they don't win.

I have a small story about rejection, an example. I was out one sunny day recently and had a coffee and muffin. I sat down and noticed a couple ladies I knew at the next table. One of them said 'oh hi'. I said politely 'hi'. One of these people used to be an art agent for me as I temporarily hired them but eventually let them go as they were more interested in promoting themselves than me. This woman thought she was high society, high in the nose, as she once dated a lawyer and bragged about it. It was this very woman who rejected seeing me, she rushed away with the other lady as they picked up their lunch and left, she looked at me as she left and said 'what are you eating, oh a muffin' and smirked. I didn't

care. I thought oh well she can't handle seeing me and must run away. It felt like grade school when you sit beside someone and they get up with their buddy and leave. Sheesh.
So I could let her make me feel less of myself and that I got rejected and feel self hate and let her feed my demons. But I didn't. I just thought oh she has problems. (which she does). I felt compassion and empathy for her. It was sweet justice as I saw her the next day working at a store I frequent. She was lowest on the totem pole and making minimum wage. Who was the confident one now? She said hi when she saw me and I was kind, said good for you, congrats on the new job and change is good. She agreed. I showed her love and compassion. But deep inside I felt yah she doesn't love herself and powers on being above others. She said 'wow saw you twice in a row, yesterday and today'. I just replied, 'yah lucky you!'. She didn't expect that or know what to say. It was real funny.

I know who I am and how I serve the community and others and my career, passions and abilities. I also know how much I love and respect myself and won't let anyone tinker with that. Try as they may. So be strong, love yourself under all circumstances, big or small.

SADNESS AND GRIEF

We all need to embrace and share sadness. As with any load, it is better carried with the help of others. Don't be afraid to say
' I feel sad today'. We all have those days, it is only temporary. If you find yourself telling you and others this alot though, you may need professional help and /or medication to get out of the funk as it may be a chemical imbalance vs. simply the 'blues'.
When you open up to those you trust, they should be kind, understanding and supportive, otherwise it is not a true relationship and you should move on. Every relationship I feel has an endpoint, be it a job, friendship, maybe even marriage. We all

know when we are there. Don't be afraid or too shy to find someone who truly cares. Keep searching if you must, til you find one who'll listen, even if paid to. We all need a helping hand, like a team or running a farm, it takes many, many who are, or act like family. There is nothing to be embarrassed about or looking "weak" when we present to others we are having a bad day or don't feel quite right.

In vulnerability there is only bravery, remember this. Me myself, I am very open and will share when appropriate some of my deepest concerns whether for me or for others. If people want to judge or talk behind my back, it certainly says more about them and their fears then it does me and my fears. "When one door closes, another opens, just keep knocking."

If we can't be heard or understood, it tears us apart and I've already discussed rejection and it's implications. Don't be quick to judge and reject people, if you feel something about someone negative, go look in the mirror and say to yourself "now am I perfect"?..... "do I not have any problems?" If you say yes your perfect then by all means go ahead and judge, as you are one in a billion . If you say you have 'no problems', then you are just lying to yourself and maybe others. We all have our good days and our bad. Our good days help us get thru the bad and sometimes our bad make us feel better about our good (more appreciative). Much empathy and compassion can be gleaned from feeling sad and sharing with others. It can help build more trust and stronger relationships. Rarely will it destroy them, unless this person you tell is downright cruel. So like me, say to yourself "what have I got to lose telling someone how I feel." Surely I will release it and save myself. Surely they may be strong and having a good day and help me carry my burden(s).

Pride is not in staying quiet or keep to ones self ones sadness. That is not being strong. Even recluse people need to share. We are strong and courageous when we step up and say this is how I

really feel whether accepted or not. Be able to handle the results, take a risk and trust. 'We cannot be fearful and trust at the same time'. Win yourself in the end and your sanity.
So take a chance, just like the lottery, learn to trust and believe in people, even with your most intimate thoughts and problems, you may be pleasantly surprised how they say "same with me"!**We are never alone. Feel good you asked for help.**

THOSE ON DISABILITY

Some people I understand who have fibro are on disability.
So many people feel guilty and insecure about their situ of being on disability- embarrassed. Don't be. Be happy and proud it exists for you, a support, a crutch for when you need it. It is not forever remember and we all go thru "stuff". If you truly want to be off the crutch you can, you can help regain your health by implementing my methods and knowledge, go back to work and eventually be 'off disability' for good. It is hard on the self - esteem to be on it long term, it's easy to just get "lazy" and feel entitled and fail then to contribute like you can. Always use your time wisely, no matter how or when given in life. Make yourself useful. Don't waste time. And only tell a small few (if need to) you trust that you are on disability as people tend to judge, but not all , nor always. Some have great compassion. It is after all a pension so use it and be thankful, some countries don't have any programs when you get sick, instead you lose your independence and live with relatives. So be grateful and quiet and determined.
A Fact: Disability can keep you down and discouraged. I know of someone we'll call him "Arthur", he tried desperately to get off disability so went back to school (struggled with funding) so he could try to work. He worked, system took his money (deducted cheque) and on top of this, he now had debts to pay. While they took all his money, he later became injured (with no savings now) and he is now worse off than when he began his journey to

improve his life and get off disability. They give no incentive for one to work, always watching the money made and deducting, so the money can go back into the pockets of big govt (they need their pay raises and lunches!). In some provinces one may keep all they make and save it (Alberta, not BC).

The system simply does not give any incentive or encourage or push you to help yourself and better your life. It feels like true punishment for being ill is what Arthur says. They do NOT distinguish between disability and welfare, making it the same amount, same pay schedule and same rules, when completely different circumstances. They could not be anymore totally different disability and welfare. It's time govt. change it and start encouraging people vs. put under their thumb and discourage or hurt people (punish them for working).

SELF WORTH

What is self -worth? Well it is the way you feel about yourself, view yourself and value yourself.

Self Worth very much impacts ones' thinking, emotions and thus behaviour, all entailing ones resultant personality.
Some self worth can be genetic, some environment and some due to abuse endured. Abused people have a real problem with self worth because they have more of, and more often, these bad demons in their head. Always putting them down and being self critical. Perhaps a memory or voice from the past (whether a parent, friend or teacher) repeating itself in the persons brain over and over.
One needs to rebuild themselves up and seek psychotherapy to squash these negative voices. You can turn these negative thoughts into positive by feeding yourself NEW positive ones and REWIRING the brain so to say (called neuro-plasticity). One can read plenty of books on self- esteem and self worth etc, but

basically you have to get in and do the hard work by rewiring your brain. Books can act as helpful guides but really professionals are the way to go (plus yourself). You can do alot to improve your self – esteem and self -worth so it can change, don't worry. Alot of people muffle these (demon) voices with addiction, say drugs or alcohol , etc. This is not preferable as it is a form of not "confronting these demons", just as you would an enemy, say if someone strange and mean walked into your house and started berating you. You would confront and deal with it. Same thing here. **You CAN feel good about yourself again.**

So many people especially nowadays have such low self worth and low self esteem as expectations of a "perfect life", like the "jones", just keeps getting drilled into our heads. We feel inadequate by not having a cell phone or the best newest computer nowadays, something so insignificant and really petty to get worried about. Be who you are, with what you've got, on your own individual journey (path) in life. As you stray from the mainstream and do more what pleases you, not others, you will come to find self confidence and self reassurance leading to more self worth. March to the beat of you own drum so you only have your 'self imposed expectations' to meet and follow vs. the "neighbour" or media imposed expectations (marketing telling us what we need). Honour who you truly are and your strengths and ability to grow and change, to improve and move forward.
Take steps everyday to improve your self -worth. Feed yourself respectful, congratulatory words in meditating, like a parent encouraging you. Be a parent to the child still deep inside of you.

Gradually the more you meditate and feed yourself more and more of these good nourishing thoughts they will eventually outnumber the bad ones and you can get a grip. Self worth perpetuates more self worth so keep the cycle going. Sometimes we can never let go of the putdowns we put ourselves thru but you can work to soften their voice and make them less powerful and overwhelming.

When you get stronger physically, as the brain is also an organ, your brain will too improve and this will all get easier as you work on your physical with the mental, they go together for there are "no borders" with the body, esp not the neck which separates visually the head from the body but they so function as one. It is all **ONE**.

As one perpetuates more self worth, the body and mind can be more calm and thus repair. You'll sleep better, you will feel more energy rather than always physically and mentally defeated. You will become a "winner" thinker. This will all be empowering and motivate you more to move forward and out of illness and into health. Strength will come back, pain hopefully dissipate and your stress levels will come down as you have now become gentler and more positive towards yourself. You'll feel more self control too, like others (including your demons) can no longer push you around. You are becoming a strong and assertive person.

So to help meditate and achieve all this, write down EVERY DAY for at least one week 10 positive things about yourself and 10 things you are thankful for in your life (easy)-could be as simple as a roof over your head or bed to sleep in or the coffee you enjoyed that day along with food! By the end of a week you should have a long list, go thru this list frequently BEFORE BED and when you wake up. You will look forward to waking up and starting your day, and you will look forward to meditating on the words at night. It helps calm the mind at bedtime, ease stress and distracts the mind off worries and headaches of the day. These words may change say every 6 months, but practice them over and over and as many attest *"we become what we think"*.

Feed yourself this "diet of words" just as you would food for your body (nourishment) and like exercise. Be disciplined. This is the hard work you must do. **Think always not where you are, but how far you've come and where your headed.**

"We dictate our destiny and future by the thoughts we think today"

SO start thinking positive and be kind to others, they'll be more likely to pay you compliments and encourage this new positive self thinking.

Your friends and family may notice a change in you over time before you do as eventually it will start to feel natural to you to treat yourself well and gentle. Treat yourself as you would if you were a small, innocent, growing, learning child. Have the same compassion, empathy and forgiveness for mistakes if they happen. Don't be hard on yourself.
Self worth is a lifelong process, to some it comes automatic but for most, we have to work at it daily.
When one seems "entitled", maybe they are just living a life full of 'faith', don't judge.

"Don't expect anyone to treat you better than you treat yourself"

As you treat yourself better and with more kind respect so will others, as you will project this new self worth. We all seem to value at a level due to what self worth is projected, for example just as you pick out a high priced piece of clothing and give respect (the higher the price, the more respect) vs. if you picked up a shirt that cost 5 dollars.
You put your own price on you! (your self value)

Self worth helps heal the body. Just look at 100 year olds, they often have a lot of self worth, and love that they are that old (proud).

Treat yourself as you would a new best friend as you deserve it. Good will come.

In conclusion, Watch what you say (speak) too as speaking it out loud gives it power and it will materialize. Never put yourself down (we all do), bring yourself up, predict a beautiful, great and healthy future for yourself.

"We can't have fear and trust at the same time"

Don't let fear get in the way of your dreams. Instead have trust they will happen and that you will be happy and healthy.
Say the things out loud that you wish to happen as though they already have. And like with magic and luck it will eventually come to be.

"Know what you deserve and don't settle for less"

"Don't live a life of entitlement but rather one of faith"
(jemma)

"Don't let people tell you <u>who you are</u> or determine your value"

"Live an authentic and honest life"

DESTINY:

Take hints in life. Took me a long time to learn this one.- people tell you things, show you things, share their experiences. All signs and signals. When we pay attention and listen we go in the right direction, our destiny. Let destiny guide you, less frustrating. Listen to your instincts both with people and situations, and yourself. Your gut is actually your second brain (it produces 90% of serotonin)- when your gut feels twisted and solid, you do not have a good feeling about something, listen to it. Whenever I don't listen to my gut instinct, I make mistakes, some big, some small, it'll happen as a billion and one things happen throughout our lives that we make decisions on. Don't beat yourself up or have regrets when a mistake happens where you did not listen to your gut. It is a natural thing to try to ignore it and want to "see" things instead of "feel". So let it go- no ones perfect. Think of all the times you did listen to it and how it helped you . Focus on the positive always.

Many things will occur that will show you your destiny so with your ears, eyes and soul, keep them all open and LISTEN- take a hint!

Trust me luck will then seem to come.

RELATIONSHIPS ARE LIKE PLAYING LOTTO 649

Relationships are like playing lotto 649, we have to gamble on people-our chances of it paying off are better than with the lottery and money.

Why is it we don't take a chance, invest a little in people who are important to us and see what happens? We play numbers and they never match, yet we keep on playing sometimes the same numbers over and over . We believe in 'winning' and hitting the big one. Why can't we just simply apply this to people in our lives?   Is it so hard?

People have trouble trusting and being open and really connecting. We live in such a disconnected world now with internet and all . Bullying and cyber bullying is at an all time high and our compassion and empathy at an all time low. We live with too many rules now, every one is paranoid, stressed out and ill. We all have them, those self critical little voices in our head which some people read as thoughts but I call them demons, because they can be so destructive and negative and mean, Bullies feed these negative voices, making them louder and louder til the person cannot stand it anymore. **Slow** bullying and torment and gossip (negative talk) can be just as damaging and destructive. No matter the bullying , hard hitting or slow, it is all the same, and we all suffer somehow. Don't let it make you suffer. If you find you are in a "toxic" relationship and it feels harmful rather than helpful, get out, blood or just friend. Save yourself. You are too valuable. It is the other persons (bully) problem to deal with and you cannot take it so personal. It'll eat you up inside and you will find yourself living according to their control and standards, not your own. Be content and happy within yourself and above all, be strong and believe tomorrow is a new and better day. Always be optimistic and give people chances but not to the detriment of yourself, your dignity and integrity. **Stand by who are you and who you want to be**. Don't let people destroy you, cause if you give them an inch they'll take a mile and crush you like a bug- it empowers them, gives them momentary self-esteem they lack.

Some people will try to control others with money, don't allow this to happen, it will destroy your self esteem. People have to trust and give people in their lives the benefit of the doubt. Maybe they are mentally ill and don't intend to say or do something- give them some slack and a break. Learn to see the positive in all and you'll live a much happier life and impact those around you with your infectious positivity. Try to help others but recognize your and their limits. Share, learn this, it will help make you happy and strong. Share, especially money. People sometimes just need a little help. Maybe for awhile. Help them out. Maybe you are all they have.

Above all, don't judge, rather try to put yourself in their shoes, imagine how they feel, what they are going thru. Especially people with mental illness, as there exists no stronger destroyer of good health. They say what doesn't kill you makes you stronger which is often true if you can come out the other side of it. When you are deep though, it is the last thing you want to hear. Sounds cliche, too cliche and meaningless. At the time you are in the dark deep hole, you need an ear, a shoulder to lean on. Help by listening, understanding. We all hate rejection, we all have a deep desire to feel connected and loved. A hug does this. Energy transfer. Giving and sharing. If you don't understand someone, just give them a hug, it won't hurt. Everything is temporary in life and we all fall victim to ruts. Just remain stronger, persevere and know you are better than what it's doing to you. It is so important we see things as "temporary". Everything goes away or comes. Don't take anything for granted. Embrace sadness like you would happiness. It is is yin and yang, we are meant to feel all- not 'just' happiness, that does not exist. It is just pure fantasy and non existent. But be there for people thru the good and bad, thick and thin. Be trustworthy and vulnerable. Show you genuinely care about the person and what they suffer, that is how we really connect.

Keep gambling on a winning relationship with others.

WATER: (we need alot)

For water is the most important thing you put into your body, drink good water. Either buy mineral water if you can afford it or get a Brita for the fridge or a Brita for your tap (change once every year or so) . This will filter pollutants out of your water and make it more healthy and tolerable (palatable). I knew when I had fibro real bad, I didn't even like to drink water (I thought surely something was wrong with me!)- I think I was just sensitive to what was lurking in it. Staying hydrated is vital to good health as it assists the body in ridding toxins from the body whether environmental or diet wise. It also keeps the blood volume up in the body ensuring good blood pressure (get o2 to brain).

Our water is certainly not like it used to be with so much ground water contamination etc, occurring. The best water may just be from a well itself or from a natural spring. I try to drink at least 1 litre/day with my most consumption during the afternoon as I run around and do things. A little before bed to assist the body helps I find too. I personally use a filter on my tap- put in glass bottles (not plastic- phytoestrogens from and BPA's- screw up hormones) and then refrigerate it. Cooler water just tastes better and I think it ups your metabolism to drink cold water. I keep at least 5-6 bottles in the fridge at all times so I never run low. Gerolsteiner is one of my favourite mineral waters and I reuse the glass bottles with my filtered water. Knowing I go thru one a day ensures I get my litre/day. Easy guide and measure.

PACING OURSELVES:
(Why we burn out after a good day)

One lady with fibro asked me why it is that we burn out. We are tired for a few days, then when we have a good day and do alot of things - wham- back in bed with a few bad days again to follow. I told her I have some ideas on why this is and here I will share them with you.

So, we all have a "to do" list, right? Well, with fibro we all have bad days and it seems to put us behind. So after resting and listening to your body, taking it easy we feel rested and energetic on a good day and then we attempt to do all on the to do list to catch up or we go out and exercise too hard. We tend to overdo it. This can tax the body and stress it as we expend too much energy we have in our reserves. Our stress levels (even positive stress) goes up and so does our adrenalin and cortisol. Our adrenals take a beating, they get exhausted as do our brain and our muscles. I believe a person with fibro has more sensitive adrenals then an average person so this is why it hits them so much harder. If you exercise too much on a good day you can deplete the muscles of

blood and oxygen and maybe 'tear' them (as muscles do), causing damage and this leads to resultant pain. The vessels become ischemic once again, no more blood and oxygen resulting in pain too. Alot may have to do with diet on a good day too.
I cannot identify exactly what happens but I know the secret is in pacing oneself- on a good day, limit your activity level to mild exertion, not medium or high. Do yoga vs. jog. Be easy on yourself.

Save your energy like you would gas in your car. Use a little at a time- don't use your full tank! I attempt to pace myself by doing one important errand a day only. Not 3-5 of them. Then I intersperse with a little tidying up and cleaning and cooking. And on low energy days I try to eat more simple like leftovers, let the cleaning go for a couple days and not do too much. I gotta say I can go full steam ahead now tho after about 3-6 months of healing and you can too. I get up at 5 am, with a good sleep, go til about 9-10 pm at nite (sometimes only 8 pm if tired). I listen to my body and what it needs, don't push beyond limits. If I need a nap in the afternoon I will take one, a small or big one depending (1/2 hour to 2 hours). (90 minutes is a full sleep cycle)

Sunday is my precious day, just for me- I shut out the phone and the "to do" list. Do things I enjoy and mainly focus on relaxing, resting, napping, reading a little or creating. This ensures a good week ahead as I go full steam on Monday and maybe peeter out by Friday. Wed I try to take naps to catch up on body repair. I really don't feel any aches or pain anymore and have bountiful energy. Sometimes Off the charts! I think my gut is in far better condition and I am getting more nutrients esp from my vitamins, of which used to probably just go right thru me - with a ruined gut. The inflammation seems non- existent now. The only time I may ache is after alot of gluten but I just combat this with 350-400 mg Mg to rid pain, it blocks the pain receptors and relaxes muscles and joints and gives me needed energy back.

Try to schedule your life as best you can while still making time for friends as they need you as much as you need them. Make time to play and enjoy a passion whether it be singing, enjoy your pet, writing, painting, swimming, biking, etc. But above all practice your health everyday- you gotta work to get it back. Always keep in your mind did I eat OK today, hydrate, take vitamins, rest, exercise (walk/ yoga) meditate (feed myself healthy positive thoughts), was I productive while at the same time taking care of myself?

I know my pet has played a vital role in my health. He keeps me calm and even, as he is really mellow and such a cuddler- he loves to love. So go ahead express love every day whether for a friend, spouse, pet or yourself. Try not to dwell on negative things or the past or past traumas, feel deal and heal. Spend alot of energy healing. The body is capable of coming back 100% I believe and stay optimistic that you can get your healthy self back, to be cured once and for all. All you have to do is treat your body, mind and spirit well like you would an engine or a best friend or a pet. We all want quality in life not just quantity so get your health back and enjoy life again- look forward to the day you'll work again- in the meantime with time on your hands and one step at a time, learn a new skill, one that puts you ahead in life and/or helps others. Contribute to this lovely world who needs you as much as you need it. Above all - pace yourself and don't take on more than you can handle.

LIFE IS A CANVAS

Life is a blank canvas where we all paint our own destiny. We often have choices, what colours to make and how it will look and how others will see it. Some people use broad strokes and bright colours and some are more subtle and subdued and perhaps even boring. However, you live your life or paint your future as it is your own, original and individual. No ones looks the same either and sometimes we even paint over it several times to get it right or due to change.

I have two friends we will call them Patricia and Priscilla. They are both so pessimistic and negative it drives me nuts. It can also be so contagious, so I take them in small doses so I don't get "infected" with it. Obviously both of them are physically ill and in bad shape. One of them, Priscilla, always has a certain whine to her voice and always has a complaint about how she feels and how life is. She has a beautiful home, a husband, few friends but is retired and NO hobbies. She is so bored, she has all this time to focus on the negative and lets face it, as we all get older the world and what happens to us seems to just get more negative (we lose youthful health and spirit). We need to occupy our time right and do things that inspire us and make us happy. Idle time is dangerous. Create hobbies if you must, do something with yourself, don't waste time, especially feeling sorry for yourself and become so narcissistic (not seeing beyond yourself)- volunteer for animals, the downtrodden or the hungry (always those in need of help).

Then there is Patricia, man she complains and is so darn negative 'about everything'. Especially those things she can't control such as all the chaos in the world, etc. I try so hard to turn her thinking onto positive and turn off her negativity but is alot of work. People get stuck in habits and negative thinking can become a bad habit. This lady is extremely ill with one illness coming after another. She is also retired with no hobbies and no friends and alot of time. If you have too much time on your hands and are a negative thinker, your bound to really sink your own ship and suffer while doing so. It never hurt anyone to think positive or optimistic even if they lie to themselves. They eventually climb out of any hole life has served them by being this way . Positive. _We create our own realities and paint our own pictures on the canvas of life._ Make sure yours is one that inspires others or looks joyful, like a beautiful garden full of goodwill and doings and alot of friends. Don't paint a dark and gloomy picture full of pain and despair. No one admires or appreciates that and it is so very sad to look at or reflect upon. Patricia can't wait to die and it is so very obvious by the way she lives. I feel for her bad habit.

There is also this woman who works a govt. job, is a receptionist (who should be nice!) and boy is she ever miserable, seems like she is serving a life sentence of some sort, I think people in jail are happier than her. Granted, it can just be her brain or personality but at least wear a smile and be a little nice to people, shoot you have a job with the govt, meaning security and good pay. I don't like when I see her at all, she brings me down. Her negativity is contagious.

We have two choices- live a joyful, happy, content, fulfilling life full of satisfaction and love, or live one full of pain, suffering, challenges, misery and no hope (alot of illness in this one – physical and mental) Make a choice and if you have to repaint your canvas, make it one people will admire and look at and say – "wow, how beautiful he/she lived their life and look what they left behind for us to cherish and enjoy!" Be all you can be, to yourself and others!

" Precisely what we think Today, Tomorrow will bring "
(jemma)

SUFFERING:

I believe quite strongly the reason we are here on earth with our gifts is to share them, help alleviate pain and suffering of others (even if just only one person) and to learn lessons on our journey. Yes, earth is a place many suffer and no one is immune. Much insight and compassion can be gleaned from the experience of suffering, which we see as so negative. We suffer because perhaps we are not paying attention and head in the wrong direction for a spell, making bad decisions which often leads to regret (more suffering). Suffering is an indicator we are doing something wrong in life whether diet, stress, relationships, attitudes, wrong decisions, reactions to others, jealousy, jobs, etc.

Suffering is a signal to change direction. And by suffering and coming out of it successfully by the changes we make whether physical, mental or spiritual, we can then become a coach, a teacher, and help others with their suffering. Just as I got fibro and suffered, found solutions, am on the right path as I am now sharing my good fortune of solutions and understanding on the topic in order to help alleviate others suffering and pain, to contribute to society. I have learned my lessons from suffering and had much time for reflection. We reflect to see if we made the right decisions and how we would have done things differently or said different things.

Some people get stuck in regret and suffering, move on I say, . move forward, we all make mistakes and the only failing is in not trying. You tried, it didn`t work, so what, try something different, maybe a different path. Let it go- no ones perfect in behaviour or actions. Forgive yourself or others if you need to and love yourself enough to not suffer anymore. There are plenty of people and resources out there now to serve as guides and problem solvers that if you reach out and wish to not suffer anymore, you won`t. There are many smart, kind, loving, insightful and wise people out there hoping to share what they know or have learned on their journeys.

Suffering I believe too, is only temporary, sometimes like in abuse esp emotional abuse, it feels like deep scars that will never heal and lives within us- try to do something with that, like treat others how you`d like to be treated. Volunteer for those abused. Write in a journal or write a book for both therapy and to share and be useful, **turn pain into purpose**. Eventually I believe those scars will heal and likely not even be a memory- you will make new loving connections in your brain and re-route all that negativity and scars to die off. A process for sure. It all takes consciousness and hard work and self awareness. To build new connections, whenever your mind goes to bad memories, replace it quickly with a good thought or memories: out populate them. Sooner or later hopefully without being fed , bad memories will die off.

And just like suffering is temporary, so can be the good times and feeling healthy, so never take these things for granted just live in the moment with them, sharing and learning and spreading joy. When you feel healthier, you will gain optimism and better control over your brain to make you more present.

" we can get so comfortable with pain, we get stuck in suffering"
"we don't have to"

(Jemma)

WORKING AND HOW WE TREAT THE DISABLED

I am so very tired of hearing people complain about working, do they really know how it feels to not be able to work and make an income?
If you don't value your job and the ability to work then do something different. If you don't like who you work for, find another job elsewhere. Pretty simple. Value working and what it gives you besides opportunity, self- esteem, experience, money, it helps you contribute to society. Every job is important and attitude often cannot be taught.

How we treat the disabled in society is disgusting and I don't mean just those in a wheelchair but for those we don't see it-mainly mentally disabled or Rheumatoid arthritis or fibromyalgia people. We need to help employ these valuable citizens and help accommodate them so they can become and remain gainfully employed. Working means so much and has greater value to a person once it has been taken away.

Employers should hire more disabled people and ask of their employees, how can I help you be the best you can be? It is atrocious how some employers, upon learning their employee is disabled treats them differently, doesn't accommodate them or will look for a way to make them quit or outright fire them. Employers may even contravene an accommodation for a disabled employee (against Human Rights) and try to get away with it by lying. These types of employers deserve no respect and must have no dignity.
It is well within your rights as a disabled employee to ask for and receive accommodations so you may work.

On the other hand, there are some employers who have great compassion and understanding and want to help others besides themselves. Theses employers are to be celebrated and recognized. What they add to a disabled persons life by giving them a job is beyond just a pay cheque. This person feels great because they can contribute and live out their passions. Often they certainly have a better attitude towards work and doing your best and are often more reliable employees. I've heard of stories where disabled people actually outperform their colleagues, even those with more experience and in a difficult job too.

Treatment of disabled people, whether working for you or not, should be that of great respect and value their worth. They may have other skills, talents or attributes far beyond others.
Above all treat people with compassion, how would you feel if you were in their shoes? Don't add to their grief, lend a helping hand or kind words. We are all here to work hard and be celebrated as individuals.

I heard an awful story concerning how a bank treated a disabled woman who was working.
They judged her, so they cussed her out, verbally attacked her, over charged her NSF (once on purpose) and kicked her out of their bank. They lacked insight and compassion and this is a horrible indicator of their lack of dignity in how they treat the weakest in the community. One lady at the bank even reported her EI to the Pension people, trying to get her into trouble. Why?, her motive, probably jealousy, insecurity and plain meanness (she was old, very overwt., unattractive and mean- the disabled woman was beautiful, young and confident) It got so messy the disabled person left their so called 'services'. She found a bank that treated her with the respect she deserved. Horrible example of how people can be to the disabled.

THE HEART

An easy test to see if you are at risk for an early heart attack is if you can touch your toes. If you cannot, it indicates that your arteries are too stiff.
Also signs of plaque buildup are:
Cold feet, hair loss and painful calves when walking.

HEART FAILURE/HEART DISEASE
It is real bad to have belly fat for the heart. The blood vessels of the body are so important and one can easily have Calcium plaque damage of the aorta (pumps blood from heart to body). Two main indicators involved in heart disease is hardening of the arteries and high blood pressure. High blood pressure damages the arteries. Hardening of the arteries helps cause high blood pressure. They are interrelated. Magnesium helps lower blood pressure, helps open the arteries and soften them. Calcium buildup makes arteries stiff and contracting. One can get too much Ca buildup if not enough Mg in the diet to keep the Ca in liquid form and going to where it is needed.

An enlarged heart can lead to heart disease.
One gets an enlarged heart if:
- Thyroid and Blood Pressure issues
- Hormone problems
- Infections

Your heart will only grow so big, then it will stop.

A good measure (better than BMI) to help determine your risk of heart disease is a waist to hip ratio:

$\dfrac{\text{waist}}{\text{hip}}$ = below .85 is good   ie. $\dfrac{30 \text{ inches}}{36 \text{ inches}}$ = .83 (ok)

This is more reliable than BMI.

Your **pulse** should be between 60-80 beats/minute ; over 90 is not a good sign. Seek help then. You can take your own pulse by lightly feeling your wrist and counting to 10 seconds and times by 6 to equal #/ minute. This is your heart rate.

For Heart Health one should have their CRP measured (blood test).
CRP measures inflammation in the body. Inflammation in the body is akin to a "raging fire" with

high inflammation = increased plaque to sooth area of inflammation

If your CRP is: lower than 1 = ideal
                  1-3 = average
                  greater than 3 = higher risk of heart attack

Autoimmune disease can up your risk.

If you get migraine headaches with aura, this is called the 2nd strongest risk factor for heart attack.
This makes sense because there are blood vessels in the brain similar to the heart and if constricted, whether plaque or blood

pressure, then a headache. Mg helps relieve this, but still get checked out.

Insomnia (approx. 31 million Americans or 10% have) and **Psoriasis** increase your risk.
Insomnia is defined as 3 nights/week less than 6 hours sleep. If problem with sleeping, leads to:

decreased immunity = incr. Inflam. = incr. Closed arteries.

Psoriasis on the skin indicates inflammation in the body and is a sure sign something is wrong. (body attacking itself). Body attacks the skin, afterall the skin is an organ. Psoriasis is an inflammatory skin condition. The immune system is attacking the skin- under surface of skin there is a war going on.
If this is happening to your skin, just imagine your heart. Immune cells are now hyperactive- Omega 3's are good for, help.

These are 9 simple things one can do for Heart Health:

1. Omega 3's - Fish oil DHA 600 mg/day
2. COQ10 - 100 mg 2x/ day (helps with statin side effects)
3. Fiber- diet 28 grams/ day
4. Low dose aspirin- 81 mg 2x /day
5. Exercise (30 min/day)
6. Vitamin D (1000-2000 mg/day)
7. Brewers Yeast (for lowering bad cholesterol)
8. **Vitamin C helps the heart**
9. Use paper filter for coffee (helps keep cholsterol lower)

Get your Blood Pressure checked as 1 in 3 people have bad numbers.

WEIGHT LOSS

So you've gained some extra pounds being inactive....here are some quick and easy solutions to help lose those pounds (all natural)

There are 4 main "fat melters" they are:
1. **CLA** - "conjugated linoleic acid". This is a good transfat, it "burns fat" (has lower melting point) CLA is naturally found in beef (grass fed) and dairy. The body does not create it, so we must take it in. So you can take in a supplement form, when you take CLA and add to fat cells, it helps dissolve fat molecules, get rid of them.
Studies have shown an 8 % reduction in abdominal fat vs. Placebo after just 4 weeks. One woman had a 56 pound wt. Loss due to just taking CLA. Since one would have to eat alot of beef (grass fed) and dairy to get enough CLA, it is best to supplement- 3 grams/day spread out (look for in safflower oil as base). With diabetes be careful due to unknown insulin resistance activity with it.

2. **PYRUVATE**- this is in the energy cycle of the body, when sugar goes to energy. Pyruvate helps bring fat up the chain of burning it, turning it into energy. Fat cells will `shrink` in the presence of pyruvate. Results one can expect is loss of body fat and body mass index by 12%. One woman has lost 30 pounds using this. You can get it from your diet- apples- red wine- red grapes or supplement- 3 grams per day along with exercise and diet will up the metabolism.

3. **MCT**- Medium Chain Triglycerides (vs. Longchain). MCT are easier to digest, goes straight to the liver where it turns into fuel=energy.
vs. Long chain fatty acids will `clump` in the body (bad).
By getting MCT you can burn 100 calories per day which will be

3000 cal per month = 1 pound fat per month.
One woman lost 100 pounds using MCT.
Diet: Coconut Oil is your best source of MCT. 1-2 tsp per day. Replace other oils or even better in recipes with coconut oil. There is also a pill form if not enough in your diet.

4. VITAMIN C- When we have stress it shows in belly fat, one way to combat this is taking Vit C, as it neutralizes cortisol which is a stress hormone and helps create the fat. So add 1/2 tsp- 1 tsp /day of Vit C to your diet- easy to do, in powder form, glass of water or in your smoothie (2 grams/day) Vit C is water soluble, so you cannot over do it.

Vit C is good for teeth + gums+ collagen, heart, bones, immunity, wound healing, lowering cortisol, ulcers, eyes.
& (cancer prevention).

Here are a few "power combos" for Wt. Loss too:

<u>1. Vit D and Ca</u>: (need Vit D to absorb Ca- need Mg to absorb D)

This combo boosts ability to melt fat. If you are currently lacking in Ca/Vit D then you'll notice 50% greater loss in visceral fat using it.
Vit D and Ca are 2 of 4 nutrients we most lack.
Basically, Ca binds to fat and takes it out of the body.
: 1000 mg D/ 600 mg Ca/day.
Yogurt is now found to be a good wt. Loss food, one of the top foods for wt. Loss. Ca in dairy products is the reason. I don't recommend you do Ca tho if feel you don't lack it.

2. <u>Oranges and Avocados</u>: With oranges you get Vitamin C (any citrus). And as I have stated several times Vit C helps neutralize cortisol. Stress pumps out cortisol which will result in a tummy up front.

High stress = cortisol = belly fat
Vit C helps knock out cortisol of the equation.

In avocados, it is the monounsaturated fat which helps lead to loss of belly fat.

3. <u>Ginger and Matcha Iced Tea</u>:
   "fat burning and oxidation"
   Ginger is a root- spice- has thermogenic effect. (high thermal temp burns fat)
   Matcha has the whole tea leave in it so all the benefits. Has "EGCG" in it. Can result in a 4- 5% increased boost in fat burning. Matcha also contains L-THEANINE which makes you alert, awake and CALM all at the same time. Also, Capsicum (hot peppers) helps burn fat- boosts thermogenesis. : 42% more fat oxidized
   : stimulates metabolism
   Matcha is good for immunity, cardiovascular health and fat blocking. Add to smoothies or make as tea. 3X the power of regular green tea.

If you have **Diabetes + Obesity = Diabesity** then avoid:

-MSG- ie ranch dressing, crackers, cold cuts etc , in everything (addicting)

-Franken Foods- more then 5 words in ingredients you cannot pronounce. (packaged foods)

-Dairy- 60 different hormones in, "anabolic – growth hormone" Affects insulin like growth factor. Calves drink cows milk to grow!

Note: Dr. Mark Hymen of the book: "Blood Sugar -----" says it is not cholesterol in our diet that is the problem for arteries but rather SUGAR. We get 15- 25 tsp/ day.

FIBROSUCCESS

incr. ZINC = incr. TESTOSTERONE = Lower Cortisol = less fat

Adrenal support and Vit C **help combat cortisol**.

Passionflower= lower anxiety=lower fight/ flight= lower belly fat.

HORMONES:

As discussed in this book alot, Hormones are intimately connected to the brain and organs. Sometimes I feel like they are the "real Boss"of the body, directing the brain (the steering wheel). Without proper nutrition, we cannot properly create or regulate these important hormones, thus our brains and other organs end up suffering or taking a hit.

The organ which takes the most hit in women is the adrenal gland. It is responsible for regulating adrenaline/noradrenaline, cholesterol and cortisol, progesterone, Aldosterone, DHEA and thus testosterone and Estrogen. So exhausted adrenals can affect our Estrogen levels. When our Estrogen levels are up, this can inhibit thyroid function. Thus high Estrogen, low thyroid. This leads to wt. gain and fatigue and slow metabolism, etc. You can, by burning out your adrenals, affect your thyroid so you will end up with hypothyroidism. This is not fun because with hypo, everything slows down, even our thinking. Our T3 and T4 (thyroid hormones) are what keeps our engines running quite literally. Metabolism and energy are showcased by the thyroid. I have hypothyroidism and thus know it's impact. I have helped my adrenals heal so that I hope one day I will have a normal healthy thyroid again. When your thyroid is out of whack you also become very irritable, the littlest things can bother you. Self-control seems gone. It affects mood and brain. SO support your adrenals, give them a rest, you do this by taking adequate Mg to

CALM the system and thus less fight/flight (cortisol, adrenaline). This will allow adrenals to start repairing.

Then you add supplements which help stress, like B vitamins and Ashwaghanda and ginseng blend (I like INNATE). This will support repair. I believe you can get your adrenals back plus thyroid and then hopefully the brain. All organs can heal if given proper tools (nutrition). As your adrenals repair you will notice more balance in hormones and the brain. You will lose some wt. too. You cannot lose wt. with exhausted adrenals !

Since our adrenals respond to stress such as chemical stress, nutritional stress, physical stress (chronic pain or surgery), you will better be able to respond to stress with healthier adrenals.

There are many **symptoms of adrenal fatigue** as many as 20 and are listed in many books or websites.

-inability to tolerate exercise
-lowered concentration
-need coffee etc.

Some things , 8 that will help with adrenal support are quite simple to implement daily:

1. Take Mg. (you can't make any Hormones without Mg)- calms mind, rids pain; energy booster for adrenals.

2. reduce sugar intake (this is also good for the gut flora to cut back)   -alcohol has sugar!

3. increase vegetable intake (no corn or wheat- GMO'd) The vegetables will have alot of fiber which helps bowel movements (feces take out cholesterol and estrogen)

4. drink alot of WATER (takes hormones to cells, cleans toxins)-preferably filtered (as discussed previously)

5. avoid soy products (interrupts thyroid function-the synthroid)/also estrogen in soy.

6. reduce or eliminate milk in diet (no Ca imbalance).

7. practice meditation- increases mental & physical health

8. sleep well at night (help repair when cortisol levels are low and not in demand)

Mg and B6 work together to decrease estrogen for those with PMS surges.

You can tell if you are Mg deficient if:

- ** grinding teeth
- have muscle cramps
- angina
- menstrual cramps
- clenching (Ca + = contracts)
- have headaches
- need chocolate pre- period (when lowest Mg in system); chocolate has Mg in it.

So stop taking Ca supplements, we usually get enough, unless you take in proper balance with Mg 1:1.

Take essential nutrients daily:

Vit A - skin, night vision
   B -alzheimers, mind, mood, and metabolism
   C - adrenals and bones, collagen (youthful)
   D -for `SADS``- mind, and whole body excellent vitamin! need Mg to absorb tho.
   E - for PMS- lowers Estrogen.
minerals: zinc(lowers cortisol), Mg, potassium, selenium and iodine for thyroid, all used to be in vegetables but not anymore with soils being so depleted and came from soils into plants!

It has once been mentioned to me that MSM helps increase vessel size and permeability, taking toxins out and helping joint deterioration, helps regulate insulin. I personally do not take it but it might interest you as it sounds like it behaves a little like Mg.

Get OMEGA 3`s as I mention over and over.
-Fish oil (Nutrasea brand)
-burns fat
-boosts mood-helps depression
-helps heart disease (mediterrean diet)
-increases focus- mind
-req`d by brain to function optimally.
Green tea extract- lots proven in studies about health benefits, being it anticancer, anti-oxidant (anti-aging), good for stress and the mind also I believe maybe help with wt. loss.

Supposedly, Mg and B6 together boost progesterone naturally (help balance Estrogen) for PMS people. I take EPO (EVENING PRIMROSE OIL) and good multivitamin (SISU) and B5 is very important for the adrenals I`ve read.

So support your adrenals, we all need some repair, no matter the age or stress level and it will in turn assist and support the thyroid and then together, working better and optimally, with proper

FIBROSUCCESS

nutrition, you may better balance your hormones which seem to steer the brain. As lower stress helps your adrenals, the adrenals healing in turn will lower stress more. A win- win. Lower stress mostly with Mg- calm the mind / Limbic system (and calm Amygdala) Practice meditation, understand your triggers and most of all eat right and exercise if you can (sends nutrients, blood, O2 and hormones where they need to be, increases blood circulation,.... so do nice warm baths if you cannot exercise yet)

ADDICTIONS

We all have them. Whether they be uncontrolled spending, eating, drinking, smoking, too much coffee, too much exercise (adrenalin junkie), overworking, etc.
Mine personally is coffee and shopping. I have a real passion for clothes. I buy quite a bit but have learned how to control it now. Nice clothes have really benefited me tho say in interviews, etc. I also give my things (clothes) onto people who need or will appreciate them so it is dual purpose- serves me and others. Many addictions occur because when we indulge in it, it makes us feel better, an escape of sorts. Helps to escape trauma or bad feelings, often those of abuse. I know I used to shop alot when my dad was alive, he would deeply upset me so I got my high or fix from buying stuff, usually on sale, so I could buy more! He had his issues and is no longer here and I do not endure his upsetting me nor do I hang onto it, I have closure thus I shop a whole lot less, if at all. I find I don't need to. What I did with my shopping addiction is make it more difficult to get money (all in my savings acct.). So I know if I love it, I'll do the work to actually go to the bank, get the money, go back and buy it. No more impulse buying. Alot of addictions are impulses. We have trained ourselves that when we do it, whatever it may be, that we feel in turn rewarded. Whether just a high.
    The brain actually physically reacts in the neurons of the

brain "lighting up" and being stimulated. The feel good center is triggered and this forms a habit. So alot of addictions become habits. **(We don't break habits, we replace them with new ones!-hopefully healthy ones.)**

One can control or learn to stop their addictions altogether by first recognizing they have a problem with something- always buying cig's, alcohol, food, clothes esp on impulse. First is recognition, next is working to replace it with something healthier like a hobby or activity you benefit from. If reading or writing calms you, try that instead of food or cigs. I have my habit of getting a daily coffee but I do enjoy it so much and also get exercise, and coffee in moderation is actually healthy for one. Smoking on the other hand is very bad for you, esp on your heart. It is so very difficult to cut down or quit but it all starts with a plan- stick to it too. Discipline yourself, practice your plan daily. Sooner or later it will automatically become habit (a good one too). You take the steps in controlling it by making it less accessible to you- more effort involved so that induces you stopping and thinking about what it is you're about to do (and how it'll affect you). When we stop and think we can reason better. So in making it more difficult to obtain, say stashing your money, not overbuying alcohol or food, you will automatically cut down as naturally humans like things that are easy and the path of least resistance.

In controlling it, slowly cut down on, reason why you do what you do and instead of making the feelings subside with a bandaid fix or escape, rather try to deal with it. Talk it out with a friend, call someone or journal your thoughts and emotions or go out with a friend or buddy as a distraction off your self indulgence. The impulse will then dissipate hopefully and you will then begin to train your brain to not "need" this fix or high. You will feel withdrawal symptoms most certainly but just try to work thru them as they will soon pass as does your bad habit with time. So be patient and kind to yourself. Don't beat yourself up if you fall off the wagon- just pick yourself up and continue on the path you set forth.

Like fibro, eventually with discipline and hard work you will find your addictions under control and only mildly indulge on your own terms, if it truly satisfies you. If you shop alot, only buy things you truly love and feel you will use alot. If you stop and think and process say how many times you'll wear something you will make better decisions. And consider that if I buy this, I have to get rid of something else. Just like a drink, you can still drink socially, just under control and only when you truly enjoy it and savour the moment, not to escape but rather to feel joy for the moment and for times to come. I don't drink much if any at all as it does not mix well with antidepressants (still on low dose.) Alcohol is naturally a depressant and I feel sad and tired after consuming alcohol, so I just don't. Coffee on the other hand gives me a little boost, a lift, my body likes it and it does no harm. Wine, once in a while is esp beneficial for heart disease, esp red wine for men (3-5 glasses spread over a week). So whatever you deal with, recognize the problem, implement a plan and follow thru with determination and discipline, one step or one day at a time, knowing well what path you are going down. We can all change habits, just takes work, like all things worthwhile and you are worth it!

(usually it takes bottoming out to get rid of an addiction)

GET OVER IT ! (Injury and Trauma)

I have an acquaintance whereby every time we talk on the phone he sounds angry. I always feel worse after talking to him. I call him anyways, maybe in a sense I am rewarding him for bad behaviour. I have compassion for him. I sense he has some issues and problems and we have had coffee twice whereby he told me he had something in his past that still bothered him. He will answer the phone with a yell of hello and talk abruptly to me. I think to myself does he not like me?...why does he answer the phone if he doesn't like me? I feel sorry for him and wish to help but he is not very open and when someone is not open it is hard to help. I talk about my book to him and he'll ask what is your approach, how do you cure it, can you cure it, is it diet, all these questions, I just reply the book will be out soon and you can read it. It is 150 pages at least, so I cannot describe in a few sentences to you over the phone. He gets real mad, I guess his mother has fibro and he wants to help her. I see his sense of urgency and demand but it's not fair to me. He gets mad, says he's gotta go and hangs up. So rude. I think oh well, not really a good way to get a copy of my book! I want to have coffee with him and discuss what holds him back from being kind and having real friends. What is it that happened to him that he just can't let go of?..here I am a good person in his life and he just blows me off cause he is angry. He always has problems it seems.

He had injured his back and was off work for 6 months. You'd think we'd do coffee or something, but no. He did nothing in the 6 months . I asked him did you write a book in your time off?(as he is quite smart), he said no, I read a couple. Always complained about his back and made me feel like I was a burden to him. Then he hurt his foot and it was swollen and he was off work for another 3-4 months. All he talks about is that he could have died. (?) Surely I think this guy has deep core issues not dealt with and let go. He cannot move forward in life and forge ahead, build new relationships. He acts somewhat arrogant. I just think, oh just deal with it and let it go for god's sake. What a waste of time and your life. I feel indebted to him as he has helped me out a bit in the past, otherwise I would just give up on him and not call or try to just be there when he comes around. Maybe he has deep mental problems I tell myself and it is not his fault. His medications are not quite right maybe. Maybe he just doesn't want any friends? I feel sorry for him, he is middle aged, not that attractive and a bit overweight. With all this you've got to have personality and kindness to attract people, esp a mate. I think a girl broke his heart and he does not trust people. This is bad and one must just let it go or you lose future good opportunities which will fill your heart back up again. Make you happy and friendly.

I am almost at my wits end with him and think what am I getting out of this relationship except misery. I feel horrible after I talk with him. He indirectly puts me down, thinks he knows more than I do (arrogance) and keeps drilling me about my book, negatively. This I do not need I figure and is not healthy for me. So I decided I will not call him anymore, just leave him alone and when he is ready to talk I will be there. Maybe I am a friend who he can really trust, open up to and resolve his inner conflict? Gotta try with people, no? I have compassion but there are limits as to when it starts to hurt me personally and about how I feel . If it is continued it must find an endpoint, either walking away or talking about things.

Toxic relationships you have to let go even, when it comes to parents or children. If people put you down or feel negatively about you, esp your dreams, it will only drag you down and not serve you well in living your life to it's fullest.

I have so much hope for people that they eventually will come around, but in reality some never do. How does this "hanging on" serve him I think, it doesn't, it hurts him and he doesn't even realize it. What a way to live. Alot of us get caught in this trap, he is not alone, we hang on so tight to something ugly in the past that it destroys our future. If someone hurt you, deal with it, go thru the emotions, seek therapy, let it out and most importantly, let it go. As it serves in the future, only to hurt yourself and eventually those around you or who you interact with. Why is hanging onto the bad so powerful I wonder?....maybe anger is stronger than love?...for others or oneself, maybe we just find it so hard to forgive? Forgive and forget it. And if it is trauma you endured see it as making you stronger and make it serve you better, moving forward.

Note ; Apparently researchers have now found that forming bad memories takes more brain power and neurons than forming good memories, thus they have more impact on us long term and may outweigh the good. So this remains the challenge, do not let them win over the good ones.

HORMONES AND DIET

Dr. Natasha Turner has a good book out called - "The Hormone Diet". I have not read it, however, I probably should and if this chapter interests you and you are a typical women with hormone imbalance, I am sure it would be beneficial to read it.

With increased stress hormone, we suppress our thyroid.
I feel that is how I truly got hypothyroidism, stress, when I was attending school in my 40's it seemed very stressful, juggling all I had to do, not as easy as in your 20's and no bills to pay then, plus your brain works optimally before age 25. So under the stress I got hypothyroidism, must be tied to my high level of stress hormone circulating in the body. At the time of school, I also decided to turn to buying food vs. clothes as I thought this was a better way to spend. Well the result was 40 extra pounds and alot of carb's, to give me the same high. It does not work to replace one bad habit with another bad habit.

SO IS:
your hair falling out?
have diarrhoea, bloating?
do you skip meals?
do you have belly fat?
are you irritable?
If you answered yes to most of these then your hormones are

likely out of balance and/or you may have hypothyroidism.
We are more prone to hormonal imbalance with increased age.
Also some contributing factors are:
- *stress (combat with exercise but hard when fibro)
- *toxic estrogen
- *toxic cortisol
- *toxic insulin (blood sugars- watch high glycemic index in foods (ie. carbs and OJ)

Timing of eating is important
What and when is important factor, don't skip meals. Eat one hour post rising- breakfast.
Every 3-4 hours eat, same time every day. This will lower insulin, lessen cravings, lessen belly fat. Don't eat at bedtime as it raises your body temperature.

Eat Protein:
The vagus nerve to the brain signals when it is "Full". Protein makes us feel more full than other foods. You should try to consume around 35% calories of protein to help stabilize hormones. Some proteins lowest in fat are: eggs or cottage cheese for breakfast.

-Hemp seeds, cinnamon (helps control bl. sugar levels- in coffee: 1/2 tsp or in smoothies).
-curry leaves help regulate blood sugar, helps estrogen detoxification.

I believe Dr. Turners book helps one restore Hormone Balance, the leptin, insulin and ghrenlin.

TIPS:
A good tip is to sleep naked, you cool down your body, it helps burn fat; skin cells, bone cells are helped.
Don't use heavy blankets or tight clothing.
-avoid artificial sweeteners

– Carbs: increase blood sugars (high glycemic index) and this in turn increases insulin production.
– Take iron for energy and prevent hair loss

Healthier choices are brown rice, sweet potatoes, carrots, beets, squash, rye and Quinoa.

Some good grains to consume are:

TEFF- for wraps, fills you up (very small grain)
MILLET- high Mg- good for migraines, muscles.
KAMUT- energy; high protein, omega 3's
BUCKWHEAT- gluten helps circulation (pancakes- Kasha) (some gluten is ok!)

for stress- use lemon balm, acts like valium.
Anti- inflammatory foods like QUINOA, are very good.

EAT:

Kale- anti-plaques, anti hard arteries.
Brocolli- anti-tumor
chicken- good for metabolism (B vits.)
-try to eat meat and vegetables together.

THE BRAIN

Copper, Iron and Zinc, these all can accumulate in the brain causing plaques.
Zinc is needed for nerve transmission and very important as is folic acid but one must watch how much zinc they actually ingest.

We Need:
- VIT E   - your plate should be: fruit/ veg/legumes/grains
- B6   - help protect memory (beans and rice)
- B12   - help protect memory (almond milk)
- Folate - "foliage" : Kale, spinach, beans; *helps nerves.*

I believe strongly in **Omega 3's** for optimal brain health too.

Dr. Neil Bernard recommends one not do minerals in a multivitamin to prevent O'Ding on them. Alzhiemers is believed to be due to metal plaques, they oxidize and destroy nerves.

Male vs. Female brain:

Female:
1. more empathy and understanding : "pre-frontal cortex"
2. have appropriate worry.
3. are intuitive- gut feeling: increased connections in white matter of the brain.
4. more self control: pre-frontal, makes better decisions.
5. more collaboration: limbic system, bonding, connectiveness.

Women make great leaders.

**Females also have (due to increased brain activity):
higher anxiety, higher depression, higher insomnia.**

To boost your mood many recommend "SAMe"- for low energy, sadness.
I tried this but did not find alot of success with, you may be different. It is stimulating - 400- 800 mg/2x day-not close to nite time. **I myself use Vit D.**

To help relieve stress- **L-theanine (is in Green tea)**
      200 mg 2-3x/ day.

Stress shrinks our memory.

"To Increase Focus"- Rhodiola (adaptogen) help with focus: increases blood flow to brain, increases longevity. 100-200 mg 1-2 x/day.

Feel and Look **Younger** with **Grape Seed Extract**: antioxidant and increases collagen (youthful).
*skin (face) health reflects Brain Health. **skin=brain**.
stress: increases inflammation which decreases collagen

Mg is proven to assist with depression. Probiotics do too.

PEOPLES PERCEPTIONS OF OTHERS

"It is none of your business what others think of you"

Perceptions are just that "what we Perceive", often the furthest from the truth, that is how magic is performed!
Perceptions thus do not equal truth.

'Our Outer Personality'

What we "wear" on the outside is our outer personality, our exterior, sometimes this doesn't always reflect our "inner" personality. Like the cover of a book, looks may be somewhat deceiving. As always stated then "you cannot judge a book by it's cover". I myself am a little overweight but this does not reflect that I overeat or am lazy, rather it is medical and I try my best in managing it. So we can never always know peoples 'true' issues. Sometimes peoples inner personality outshines their outer and people learn to disregard what they see (if not shallow thinker). Sometimes peoples inner and outer match like a great outfit but this may be rare. I can think of only a couple examples where this holds true.

So don't be too quick to judge others based on their "outer" personality rather hold judgement til they reveal to you their true inner self (like reading a good book, take time). Some people even have such emotional barriers and walls, it may be difficult to see immediately or they may have low self- esteem. What we think of ourselves, even if not true, we project and people will then perceive this. Alot of people carry low self- esteem.

People always want to look a certain way (ie dress), what others would expect, so that they "fit in" or feel comfortable (too hard on the ego not to feel comfortable), it is a brave few who do not care and express themselves however they feel, they usually have quite high self esteem.

"Genetics do not determine our SPIRITS. Rather our spirits serve to provide our genetics with what they Need (ie. Strength)."
(jemma)

Cancer (you are so strong!) and Genetics

Why is it that people with cancer who are surviving it or even passed on due to it are seen as so strong vs. someone with mental disorder is seen as so weak?
In reality it is often the mental one (who may also suffer a physical ailment and disease) who is the stronger one. Cancer, tho not cured, has so much support, money and answers. When you tell someone you suffer cancer they respond with a warm and loving hug and encouraging words like "you are so brave", "you'll get thru it", "we will help you". Why is it tho when we disclose mental illness that people look in disgust and disbelief, like you've done something wrong and they should now be scared of you and actually pull away in body language, and emotionally, abandoning you. Full of fear and judgement. This all based on past experience or rather lack of experience, or mostly media and plain old stigma. When will we get to the time where we say "oh I am

sorry", give them a hug and say "if there is anything you need I am here for you, you are not alone". When will we treat cancer and mental illness with the same respect they both so deserve?

We need to change our perceptions from:
crazy= loser, weak   to   crazy= strong, successful
   (dis-value)   (value)

I had coffee with a friend of mine and we talked about mental illness. She deals with it, as does her husband. Her husband and her have yet to tell their early teen kids about his depression for fear it will make "him appear weak, not strong like a father should be" she stated. This is sad and a strong example of stigma. They should take the opportunity to educate and teach compassion (esp for a family member) and give them personal insight. As mental illness is mainly genetic, their kids may be prone to it or go thru it likely themselves, even at a young age. Awareness is key. The sooner you help it, the better the outcome. Some children even feel and suffer from depression. Certainly, if he had say cancer or kidney disease, they would disclose.

This same friend commented how "if mental illness is all (100%) genetic and if so" then is it "not curable"? Then I gave her my point of view, which is this: if someone had light hair and sits in the sun, it will tend to go lighter, blond, as they are predisposed to being blond and the sun affects this "more" than someone who has "brown" hair (genetics). If no sun , no blonder. Sun may equate "stress" here. If avoid sun (stress) , no blond (illness), so manageable and somewhat avoidable. So we can be genetically predisposed (weakened-prone) to some disease and if the "right" (or wrong) environment to spark it presents itself, whether stress, drugs, toxicity, etc, then it can be exposed and expressed. Like cancer, it can be treated successfully with drugs and the stressors removed to manage it. Will mental illness ever be cured – no one knows, at least right now.

Ideals

Some people place their 'ideals upon others', to please and suit themselves. It makes them feel "powerful" and "comfortable"....two things humans enjoy feeling. Beauty often makes us feel comfortable (why we enjoy it so). We do not generally like ugly or disorganized things. We will try to correct it to our liking so that we feel in control and comfortable. People do not like to be uncomfortable or feel endangered (not knowing), it takes away a sense of power and control. It induces question and fear. Two things humans do not enjoy. We feel powerful in "knowing", our egos get fed. We like to know how things will be or how people will behave. If we don't sense control over these things it puts us in panic mode, like "what now"?
One of my friends is really good at placing her ideals upon me, to mold me, change me, into someone or something she feels comfortable with. Someone she can better relate to (for the most part I ignore it) Yes we impact and affect each other but it is wrong to inflict your ideals and what makes you happy and feel content upon those who are not on the same page (or have changed alot).

We all have our own individual journeys to travel and be who we are meant to be. Allow people to be who they truly are. Differences should be celebrated , not feared. It is in things being different where we learn the most and open our minds and eyes up to "new things" outside ourselves. So celebrate individuality, let people be who they are, how they want to look, the way they talk, the way they feel, even and especially the way they express.
A strong and confident person allows others to be who they truly are. Very few of us are this confident but we are out there.

"don't fear what you don't know".

Insecurities (fear, ego, jealousy)

Pets truly see us, as they are without human attributes of undo fear, ego or jealousy. We love them so much because of this, unconditional love. They reflect the best part of ourselves, which our ego enjoys. Humans have so many hangups and project their own insecurities towards others that their perceptions lack value, insight or integrity. People will perceive you as they see fit at the time, until they change their thinking, usually by new information. I know someone who was working and seen as the best worker the employer ever had until one day the worker shared a disability with them and from that time on they changed their perception (to a bad one- one filled with fear and ego). This hurt the worker immensely, to have such an earned perception change to one that lacked integrity or real basis. They now projected their ego and fears upon this person. Their new perception did not reflect now who the worker truly was, but based on their lack of compassion and lack of knowledge (fear based). So don't worry if someone does not perceive you accordingly and to the truth, it is just their hangups in the way! Some people are so stubborn in their thinking, nothing will change it. Don't put your energy into trying to change them, if they want to come around, they will, but don't sit and wait for it, move on!
Put your energy instead into those who like, encourage, and see you, for that is worth it.

People see what they want to see and what they set their mind up to see is what they will surely find- their ego dictates this. The ego craves success and being right. We all have a light and dark side and people will see the dark if they so desire or see the light if perhaps their attitude is to see the best in people. So don't worry about peoples perceptions of you, they are likely wrong and just suiting their needs or egos. What you know about yourself and how you truly are is all for you to know and only reveal if you so choose to. It takes alot of trust to reveal our weaknesses and alot of gumption to reveal our success (due to peoples jealousy). Only you walk in your own shoes, worry about your own "truth", instead of peoples "perceptions". You know your true value. In rare times people may see in us what we are incapable of seeing in ourselves, such as truth and goodness. Our self esteem (lack of) can prevent one from seeing their true worth. We all have these inner demons that put us down (esp. Artists, too self critical).

People may also form their perceptions based on their own personal power. What they have to gain if they think about you in a certain way.

The reason the way we see ourselves may differ from how other see us is due to the fact of knowledge. We all know what we are truly capable of. How can someone know all you know in a few chance meetings? Their perceptions are all guesses and assumptions based on what they look for and their own insecurities. I know of a person whereby even their own mother, who knows the person well (or should), has mis-perceptions. The mother thinks so negatively of them and places their own fears and insecurities upon them when unnecessary, if they just looked and listened and had faith. They do not know their own child, so if this can happen, then how do we expect strangers to see us as we 'truly' are?

We celebrate stars but deep down we are jealous, we put them on a pedestal only to try to knock them down. Our perception of stars are usually wrong and gossip driven, we don't truly know these people, even tho we "think" we do. Stars are often intimidating because they seem 'larger than life' and we all want to be like them (live their lives). We are all actors though on the stage of life and we project at moments what we wish to project while protecting our true selves from those who may decide to attack. So don't try to judge others (or gossip), instead keep your "own" opinions to yourself where they belong and learn to accept people good and bad, and if they show you their inner selves, celebrate the individual and the level of trust they have given you. Don't attack them, for you are not perfect!

I have an acquaintance, he changed towards me drastically after I presented a business opportunity to him. Weird. Did he get jealous, perhaps insecure? He is over sensitive. He perceives us as friends, however, I do not have any contact info for him thus we are acquaintances. He started perceiving me a certain way then I know myself and who I am. His ego drives him, the being right. He chooses to see the dark for some reason, so animosity grew as this is what he expected. Our expectations of others can come true, we just have to be determined and look for them, good or bad ones.

"Funny how we perceive ourselves is not often how others perceive us" He told me. Yes that is because we can project falsehoods; only we truly know and live with ourselves so unless someone pays your bills, don't worry about how they perceive you, they are merely projecting their fears, jealousy and egos upon you. Move towards those people in life who appreciate you, this will bring out more of your best. Only a therapist or true friend will tell us how we show ourselves to the world like a stage performance, in essence we are all on stage (not real). And nobody can perform perfectly.

People are Fluid

People are "fluid", they change (like plants- can grow/die/replant). People like to put others in "boxes", with labels. How we see, and judge and "label" has to do with our egos (knowing is feeling powerful). People are able to change and grow and others around them should learn to adapt to this change. Learn and accept the new information. What they now bring to the table vs the past. People can and will change if they want to, or sometimes have to, due to illness.

If people don't change together with each other in acceptance, then they drift apart, (why so many divorces happen I gather). Accept others for who they are, don't try to change or make them accommodate you, they are here for a reason, allow them to shine and be who they truly are.

We often put up walls in defence. Try to please others, be something we aren't. Don't worry about anyone's perception but your own, be an independent thinker and believe in yourself. Live for you only. Only you truly know who you are. For only you walk in your own footsteps, not others. Have hope and compassion for others and their quirks (or struggles)

Our egos have us put others down or criticize (power). Some things such as mental illness are not discussed, if so, we'd all see how much we share in common and have thus more compassion for each other. We deeply need more compassion in today's society where it seems 'every man for himself'. Technology has changed the way we communicate, making us more fearful to speak up as we are afraid it will go "viral". Everyone knows everyone else's business nowadays.
We have lost a sense of privacy and respect for it and in essence for ourselves.

JEALOUSY, VENGEANCE AND BEING CALLED CRAZY

(jealousy)

Women (not all-generalizing) especially over men, can easily get jealous or vengeful. Never piss a women off I always say! ...some can go for blood and often get it. Gossip is often a tool to carry out jealousy and vengeance. Deadly in some cases. Why women especially get jealous? I think it has alot to do with estrogen surges and insecurities (pressures by media) as well as them being miserable and not in a 'happy place' in life. Misery loves company as they say and if they are down and miserable they want you there with them! These people will turn on you, talk negative (toxic) about you, overwork you, do hateful things, sabotage you, whatever they can manage to do to feel they are "getting even or getting you back", (even tho you do nothing).

Their vengeance is deadly in that they won't care if you hurt so bad that you hurt yourself (either physically or emotionally). When people are mean to you, analyze INTENT , not outcome. Here you will find truth, WHY they do what they do, not what they do. "What they do" is often too complicated to analyze. "Grass is always greener", we can never truly know all aspects of someones life, just judge and perceive and often these can be misleading and not true. Things are not always how they look or appear. Sometimes women may feel threatened by you. You challenge a weak part of them with your strengths, this gets their backs up.

Happy, content, successful, confident women don't indulge in jealousy and vengeance. They can easily let things go- brush it off for they are too happy and confident to bring themselves to such a low level. That is why it is very important to be around these type of women, not unhappy ones, especially if you are super happy and successful. Be mindful who you surround yourself with so you don't end up getting stabbed in the back. Betrayal and stabbing in the back hurts especially when you don't see it coming nor deserve it in anyway. We can never know or understand always why someone does something, sometimes it is just because of plain genetics (brain wiring), the "personality" they have. Sometimes forgivable.

Being smart, beautiful, witty, hard worker, likeable, free or rich all are some factors which may induce jealousy. If a person does not feel your same level they will certainly try to bring you down to theirs. Hurt goes round and round. That is why I often just let hurt go- it ends at me. I project love in place of it as this is what I wish to circulate. You deflect hate with love and compassion. Don't allow others to bring you down to their "miserable, unhappy" level. Don't. Be strong, walk away. Ignore them. Get them out of your life if they hurt you. Protect your happiness, "Don't let anyone or anything steal your joy". Keep moving on forward without them. Rejoice in your glee and happiness and if you feel someone has hurt you (whether intentional or not) let it go as their Karma, people know what they do, don't seek vengeance, this will only come back to hurt you.

(vengeance)

Don't try to get "even" with people or teach them a lesson. If it means "justice", it will come eventually on it's own time. Getting even just hurts you and makes things worse. People know very well what they do and how they treat /hurt others, let them just live with themselves. They will endure it's KARMA. Most if not all people have consciences and memories and a sense of what is just/fair. So you don't need to step in to teach them something- they will learn on their own and often what people do , whether good or bad comes back to them 10 fold. Sure people make mistakes so they deserve benefit of the doubt. But there are also many who mean what they do for reasons unknown, often even unknown to themselves. So don't try to understand motive, intent or even people's unique personalities. When someone is really odd in personality I chalk it up to the wiring of their brains- genetics, thus not their fault or intentional. Even if someone physically attacks you (by the way words can be just as powerful/hurtful)- this action of theirs may be beyond their control (again genetics).

People best manage their personality if they know they are not perfect (and really who is?). As I've said before people have a dark and a light side and MOOD (their outlook, thoughts, perceptions) often determines and dictates which one they show, unless they have alot of "self control". So don't try to "control" peoples personalities, accept people as unique individuals with a certain hand they have been dealt (genetics, environment) and accept (think) that they are 'doing their best'. This attitude and approach lessens frustration with events that occur. *"The best one can do"* is all we should expect from others as perfection is impossible, so is going beyond what is possible for them. The world has a long ways to go in being more compassionate. If someone behaves strangely, treat them like you would someone in a wheelchair, with compassion and understanding for their shortcomings, especially if this person is honest and often apologetic. I don't ask you to take abuse from anyone, just give love in the face of frustration and be a good listener above all. Sometimes all someone wants or needs is to "be heard", listened to and respected. This is in itself very valuable and a good diffuser.

It has been shown in studies that self worth is strongly associated with depression. When we have depression we have low self worth and this can cause insecurities, more women are prone to depression than men thus the reason maybe more women suffer lower self worth and therefore these insecurities which trip them up.

"When people call you crazy"

People will often call someone crazy if they are jealous, or maybe "crazy" themselves. Crazy is an overused word and just like the word "fag" just as hurtful. We must abolish it and not use it derogatory towards others. Embrace crazy, be eccentric. Geniuses are crazy, don't ever forget that, and we all need geniuses. Rather than crazy they just have a unique and special way of thinking, like outside the box or an overactive (hardworking) brain. When someone calls me crazy (as I am an artist), I take it as a compliment I am different and unique, special, I standout, I smile and move on. I look at intent though and it tells me alot about that person and their insecurities and attitude. Embrace crazy. Just like gays embrace 'being gay'.

"Judging a person does not define who they are. It defines who you are".

"When you cease to make a contribution, you begin to die".

CLIMB THAT MOUNTAIN!

Don't ever let someone tell you that you can't do something. If it is in your heart and/or a passion, go for it. Reach for the stars. It may be a mountain to climb to get to your goal but go ahead and start up that mountain one step at a time. If you don't plan and act you won't follow thru. Don't let anyone dictate or tell you your dreams either. If you can't walk, try to prove them wrong and walk. Even against the odds. The more against the odds, the sweeter the victory, when you achieve climbing up that mountain. It won't be easy as most mountains are challenging but just like when you reach the top- there is the reward, the view (perspective) and the feeling of accomplishment and the ability to reflect on the journey it took.

I interviewed someone I believe to VERY inspiring. It follows a story of a fellow colleague, we'll call him Glen for privacy. He is a cardio tech too but hasn't always been one. In his late 20's he told me he was diagnosed with Mental Illness, it was a bad breakdown, his future looked bleak, never to be independent again. Right in the prime of his life too. I won't say what it was, just that he was bad enough to be institutionalized like put into Riverview (a psych hospital shut down for now). Not too many people in his life gave him much hope or alot of support (except the odd stranger). They kinda gave up and resigned to the fact Glen would always be ill and badly too. But Glen had a different and stronger point of view. He was determined to get better, more healthy and improve his future prospects. After much trial and error, the right medicine seemed to have been found that worked best for him. Lucky he thought. Now I can manage better and put my life back together he pondered. It was a daily struggle just getting up and doing chores and feeding himself, not a great way to live.
Glen had no social life or many friends as no one wanted to hang out with him as maybe they thought he was contagious or just plain stigma on their behalf. This didn't stop him, when he was at

his lowest, he fought the hardest, kept an optimistic attitude and did alot on his own (helping himself). He worked daily on his health, something people just take for granted and found helpful things for his brain health. He at least for the most part, had a physically functioning body and this was a plus. He could not work, no one would hire him, he did not have alot of experience.

Having gotten ill so early in life, he dropped alot of his aspirations (to work helping others), and wished to make things happen again for himself. He understood very well his disability and affliction and learned alot of compassion along the way, along with deep insights. This was a handy tool he thought. What most kept him moving forward was a good attitude- determined, optimistic and always hoping, with working hard. He tells me he wanted a better life then he was living, so decided to try to go back to school, even though he had no money for it. Well the money came for Glen, from a philanthropic organization (he had absolutely no family support). These kind strangers helped make his dreams come true. He convinced them that he could in the end get hired and use his skills, that he would not be a waste of the funding. This he told me took alot of convincing and proving himself. There was one special person who cheered him on and pulled thru on the funding for him, a real life changer he appreciatively thought.

He became a Cardio Tech just as I am. His interest was in helping others and studying psychology seemed too difficult to achieve at the time. As with his experience, he now understood alot about the brain and human nature. His cardiac studies were a struggle and no one knew of his disability, he wanted to be treated the same as everyone else. He also considered the fact people would not give him the credit he deserved if they knew of his illness. He succeeded in completing his diploma, with honours, best student in his class. He had superseded his goals. Now it was time to work and get hired. He had a tough time finding work though, something he didn't expect, the market was filled with plenty techs, alot of them younger and better looking . He felt disadvantaged but never gave up. One day a dream job happened for him. Part time and in a private setting as he could focus on developing patient skills. It was an exciting time for Glen. He finally felt successful and slightly independent for the first time in a long time. This instilled more hope. He tells me he felt like a person in a wheelchair that could walk again. He climbed that mountain.

Turns out while he was high up on that mountain there were people ready to push him off. A person at work made his life miserable. Why, because this person had very low self esteem, was insecure and themselves miserable. They needed company. This person was inherently bossy and a bully. Two things Glen had a hard time with. This person was also very unattractive and very overweight and just not happy where they were in life. Old too. Glen became this persons' target (this person was a female co-worker) She bullied him and bossed him so much he couldn't take it anymore with all he was challenged with. He was just there to work. She was probably jealous as Glen had a much more important position at work than her and this intimidated her. One day, after enough harassment he told this co-worker to please stop it. Well she didn't like that, being pointed out what she was doing and then asked to change her incorrect habits (and bully personality) No bully likes to be told they are a bully. Well she retaliated worse now, wanted Glen fired. She did a real number on him, sabotaging him at every turn. She didn't play a major role in his job except she ran a bit of the office which impacted Glen.

Glen finally had to get help from the bosses to keep working. He disclosed his disability and the ongoing bullying. He had accommodations put in place to prevent the bossy co-worker from sabotaging him. She now had limits to her evil doings. So she thought of other ways and this was to slowly torment Glen, getting the bosses on her side, poisoning Glen with gossip and poor attitudes towards him and the job he was doing. No respect.

This wore on Glen but he persevered. Did his very best and he was recognized as the best employee and best Cardio Tech his boss had ever had. A real achievement. His plan was just to work and do a job, mind you he exceeded that plan by being determined, happy, optimistic, respectful and working hard (gave 120%). It was a joyful moment in Glens life to contribute and gain such respect both for himself and from others. He actually helped save many lives and made a huge difference and impact on the patients in a very positive way. Glen tells me nearly everyone complimented him on his skills and personality and competency when he worked.

Well it was soon after he disclosed his disability that the employer changed. They were now looking for his "disability", hard too, to actually fire him, as they were judging, worried of his skills and abilities he had worked so hard to prove. They didn't care, just wanted perfection in their clinic. Compassion, sympathy and recognition went out the window and he now still had the co-worker wanting him fired. What to do? He could not quit, rather he stayed on top of that mountain and worked harder, proving himself even more. One day it became too much though, as the employer (must of wanted glen to quit) pushed him past his limits, the accommodations. It tested his disability and made it snap, like a twig that is bent continuously and too much. Glen was injured and knocked off his mountain now. Wow what happened, should Glen have given in and quit before disaster struck, NO. He did the right thing by hanging in there and doing his job even when they exceeded his limits. He did not show the snap at work, as he just went into deep depression from this point onward. Well Glen took time off work to heal as health was most important to him and the key to him being on top of that mountain. The employer was pleased, they got rid of a "disabled" worker, one with mental illness. The co-worker, needless to say felt successful (for once) and full of glee. Now she could get more prey to bully around. And she looked like the "hero" to the bosses (her plan). Glen instead of getting angry, got better and got a lawyer, as the employer tried not to give Glen his job back and even fought him on employment insurance (so he could at least eat), what was all this about Glen wondered, why hurt such a diligent and "golden" employee, was it stigma? Were they worried for and about themselves and not Glen? It was all very confusing and selfish he thought.

The employer, hating Glen so much by now, submitted a falsified ROE (record of Employment), a legal document, to Service Canada in the hopes of hurting Glen further. Service Canada delayed paying him and gave him a hard time all because they believed the employer over Hardworking and Diligent Glen. Disgraceful & Pompous attitude. It is not uncommon, the employer retaliate against an employee, Service Canada told him.

However, Glen got back up and is climbing the mountain again. He got better and is fighting to get his job, rightfully and legally his, back. He wants to work again even in spite of what happened. He is forgiving because he understands stigma and lack of compassion for the mentally ill (he doesn't like it, but understands it exists) He is now on his way back up the mountain of success and pride as he takes the employer to the Human Rights Tribunal for violating his rights to an accommodation and not being treated fairly or "just". (It was needless, him getting injured at work.) In doing this, he will one day again be on top of that mountain feeling nothing but pride and righteousness while setting an example for all who follow. He will not let them or anyone else beat him down and not treat him with the proper respect he earned and so deserves. As Glen is stronger and more determined than ever, one of the strongest people I have ever met. Inspiring....

So the moral of this story is, climb that mountain, no matter how physically or mentally hard and treacherous. Reach for the stars and your dreams and don't let anyone get in your way or make you stop. If Glen can do it, with all his obstacles and all that stigma, certainly you can too. Even when people knock you off the mountain, which will happen several times in life, you don't give up, pick yourself up, heal, get back on the horse and keep moving forward. Those who knock you down will learn their own lessons, just ignore them. Battle them if you must to make a point of who you are but only do this with a lawyer as most only respect lawyers (and they wield a mighty sword!) Fight for your rights and what is civil. Don't give up because people tell you it is the best or only way. That is called losing. Don't lose, win. Be a Winner. You have to live with yourself and you know your battles so keep on keeping on. Push til you reach your dreams and goals.

Anything is possible and by witnessing your determination and hard work, others will become inspired.

And that is a gift, to INSPIRE others!

LET'S TALK ABOUT IT:

Lets talk about depression!....today is Sept 10, 2013 called "WORLD SUICIDE PREVENTION DAY".
I was going to my pharmacist today of all days to pick up some synthroid and mentioned to him, guess what today is, he had a customer and said to me, no what day is it?....I replied, today is world suicide prevention day!....he grimaced like he was then embarrassed, he said well I guess that is something to celebrate (sarcastically), I said yes enlightenment is always good and healthy, we should all talk more about it, <u>we don't talk and people die</u>, he got too embarrassed (but agreed) and I was about to depart, said it's important people bring it out from the shadows, alot of your customers are extremely suicidal, and then I backed up and said well 'kinda' suicidal, depression is real popular. I left in disbelief that a pharmacist was even embarrassed to talk about it, like I was talking about private parts or something of that nature.

Horrible I thought, the lack of insight. Suicide remains one of the most preventable deaths of all illnesses worldwide, I am proud I had the guts to mention what the day meant, esp to my pharmacist, he is the owner too of the pharmacy.

Depression should now be discussed like we discuss cancer, it is out there, not going away and only getting worse. It touches people from the average joe to world athletes to movie stars, everyone with talent, and is a sad waste. Imagine if they could just pick up the phone before they decide and just talk openly to someone about how they feel, imagine maybe it would save them?.....just hearing someone put things into perspective or just hear them out, sort thru their feelings. It is no ones fault one feels suicidal, a chemical imbalance in the brain, like something wrong with your kidneys or heart. What is the harm in just being open and talking about how we feel, esp when down?.....that is when we really need a friend. When I told the pharmacist what day it was, I felt kinda 'low' and embarrassed with the pharmacists reaction and I have known him for 6 years. I felt like I said something inappropriate or wrong. I was in the end proud I opened a little discussion tho. One drop in the bucket.

It is not odd nor embarrassing we once in a while feel like ending it all, we all get down and blue. We are after all, all human. It is so sad when I reflect on lives lost to suicide, I forget the rates but I think one person every minute dies in the world or it maybe every 30 seconds?

I know when I get down I have people I trust and can talk it over with. It'll happen especially being an artist, we are so self critical and pick on little things. Everyone should have someone they can turn to. At least there are help lines established but this is not the same when one is in crisis mode, who wants to talk to a stranger then?.....we need someone who loves us. We all have at least one person we can rely on and say loves us. (I hope)

I am hoping one day, and I hope I see the day, that depression and how we really feel becomes everyday discussion and the importance it requires, is put properly on it. Imagine the lives it'd save. We have to stop feeling ashamed of the word "suicide" and treat it like the disease it is. How did aids ever overcome it's stigma, because people took a stand and said "this is enough, I have aids and am not ashamed!" Look at the progress we have made there, these people are now living, and full lives too. We all hit a little bump in the road but tomorrow is always a new day and as always, everything is temporary, just wait it out, call a friend, journal if you must, write a book perhaps!...let's get talking!!

One recent example of a great loss is Gia, the TV "bachlorette", she was in the midst of hanging herself, called her mom, they were talking, she took her last breath with her mother on the phone, why is it she didn`t get saved, just by words....simple, what did they talk about, did Gia feel comfortable saying what she was wanting to do. It is times like this that we can change a persons life and keep them living. Another more recent one is comedian/actor Robin Williams, a super talent we lost to this, did he have someone to turn to?
Every life is a gift to be cherished and protected.

Be a friend, even to a stranger. What will it hurt, certainly not you.
``If you can, do``, I always say.
        Lets stop letting people lose their lives, unnecessarily.

``If you have a heart, you can experience a heart problem, just as if you have a brain, you CAN experience DEPRESSION!``
                                      (jemma)

"We can all use a little more <u>Acceptance, Compassion, and Tolerance ("ACT")</u> when it comes to dealing with humans and each other"

FOOD SENSITIVITIES - why we are such an Angry nation.

Note: it has now been proven by science that 'transfats' produce aggressive and angry behaviour in people.

Foods & diet we eat are so very important, they should be left alone in their natural state as much as possible. Some of the major four foods that people are most often sensitive to are:

wheat

milk

corn

and soy.

This forms a lot of North America diets, especially wheat & milk. When we eat these foods in high quantities (some people so sensitive even a small amount affects them) than the symptoms of irritability, anger, Foggy brain, Bloating, Inflammation (pain) occur majorly. These foods are over processed and GMO'd. Our bodies don't recognize these Franken foods. Milk has way too many hormones in it too, throwing off our regular balanced hormonal cycles, etc.

We are easily stressed and very irritable if we have food sensitivities. Notice how nice and peaceful vegans and people who eat organic are. They are not destroying their body or brain with "foreign" foods. North America has gotten so angry over the past two decades, most noticeable these past 5-10 years. Mental illnesses are on the rise as people "snap", we're turning to addictions due to stress for people feeling bad (due to peoples meanness). Bullying is on the rise among teens and even co-workers as a lot of them were raised on these unbearable foods we have ingested. Stress is on the rise, people drive crazy and people simply are not polite or nice to each other anymore. Especially if you do not fit into their mold of "normal". What is happening? Peoples brains are suffering.... where's our compassion? When people get stressed let's face it, they get bitchy. Especially women. Yes it's true. We can do a lot to curb this by switching our diet and letting our brains (and because they are organs) heal. Be nicer to one another, feel more at peace, less stressed. I know my job of stress testing people should be a stressful job but it isn't- I don't feel stressed. I know what I'm doing and remember that I am part of a team at work.

How can we help North America? We can -start labeling foods as GMO'd and give people the choice of whether they want to hurt their brains or body with that food. Make people more aware. Knowledge is power. More books written about our diet and these harmful foods the better equipped we will be to make better choices. We eat cheap, that is when we get unhealthy. And the people in charge of food production are making our staples cheaper and cheaper for more profits. Our food has been too manipulated and at a high price. While health care costs skyrocket. The price we all pay.

So many people suffer unnecessarily. Key part of fibromyalgia is our diet, we have to look after our brain and body. I have covered well what one needs to do but one does not have to fall so bad you have this disease to make a change.

If we change our diet, we would all be happier as a result and more harmony in this stress filled world, if we make a change for the better.

WE ALL DO IT- WE JUDGE

We all do it-we judge especially each other. The way we look, act, dress, where we go, what we Drive, where we live. We can't help it. Our brains are wired for the negative. It serves the purpose of avoiding danger. It has been shown in studies how the brain reacts more to negative things versus positive, pleasant experiences. It is easier for us to remember, to retain this negativity. So when it comes to judging this is where negativity steps in. We pick up the negatives in a person rather than their positives. When we really focus on what we want to find(the negative) we will certainly find it as no one is perfect no matter how hard they may try. True we are all flawed. This is why it is very important to stop yourself when you can and switch gears, try to see the positive right away in people and things, the weather and situations. Makes for happier you and will affect this person being judge to a lesser degree. Don't you think perhaps people have enough problems they don't need you picking on them. Don't you think they're fully aware.

Optimally we like to judge and get in the habit of it as it makes us feel better about ourselves. We'll look at what she's wearing… certainly my clothes are nicer, more expensive. Petty meaningless things but the more insecure you are with yourself the less compassion you have and will judge. It is automatic and a bad habit. People must try cure their insecurities and not project when it comes to putting down others, see that they too are flawed and have much more work to do on themselves than say this person in jeans and a T-shirt.

We are hardest on the poor, disadvantaged and homeless as they scare us. Our negative fearful side of the brain kicking in. However, they are human too and feeling negativity towards them, they do not need nor ask for this. Don't bury a person when they are half buried themselves. Practice patience, compassion and taking in the positive in every person, place or situation, you will feel better and so will they. Again making for a better world that we live in.

SELF LOVE

Self-love is so hard to practice. So many of us look to our environment and outside factors for love. But alas, we must truly feel it within ourselves, in our hearts and most importantly our words, what we feed us as thoughts about ourselves. We all do it, are self-critical, punish ourselves with self-defeating thoughts especially when we are weakest- we must put this in check- stop the negative self sabotage and replace with positive self loving thoughts and kind words to yourself. We feed our brains just as we feed our bodies. It is bad enough we pick up on the outside world and their possible hateful and unkind words, to do this to ourselves we must stop and we do have the control and hopefully the awareness. Self-deprecating thoughts are mainly a bad habit which may form in early childhood, perhaps a hard parent or teacher. We must replace that habit with new healthy thoughts.

Encourage yourself, send yourself love, appreciate all your good qualities and how you contribute to society. Complement yourself whenever possible.

A good practice to help retrain your brain as if every night before you sleep keep a journal and you write down three to five things you appreciate about yourself-say that was nice you held that door for someone or paid someone a compliment. " Gee you are a determined and hard worker" "I value your insight, wisdom and compassion" simply a pat on the back. Say anything to yourself positive, will surely become a good habit. Eventually as you sleep with these as your last thoughts of the day, will help create the self-love. Throughout the day also tell yourself good things about yourself (encouraging). Stop expecting this love (especially unconditional) from the world and others, you will only be disappointed as so few people really do love themselves and/or go through what you do. When you have the self-love you will automatically attract better people to your life and create healthier relationships. Give yourself that unconditional love, love that inner child in you ,care for them, nurture them. Treat them as you would a small child or a best friend, be supportive not destructive or critical. You will find you set boundaries and will have respect for yourself. As you attract better people in your life this will fuel your positivity for yourself and encourage this great habit of self-love. Self-love is so very important and only helps yourself to be better in life and have a more joyful life. Don't get stuck.

Self-love takes a lot of training and effort but sooner or later it will become effortless. Just begin by stop expecting it from the outside world, it is too rare. Begin with yourself.

Live in the light, not the shadows.

WHEN OUR HEARTS BREAK OVER A LOSS
(dedicated to my dear cousin)

It hurts when we lose a loved one. This is just a fact, no matter the relationship. We are connected thru life and share experiences and maybe troubles.
So when we lose someone it hurts and our heart feels broken, a kind of ache.

Recently, I just lost my favourite cousin, she was only 35 years old but quite disabled and although it was sudden and somewhat expected, it caught everyone off guard. She did not suffer in the end, she passed in her sleep. She had brain tumours and heart problems and seizures all her life, so had it very rough here as her tool, her body, did not give her the strength she needed on earth but for what she lacked in physical she certainly made up for in spiritual. She did not judge others, was always kind, offered all a hug and said I love you at every opportunity, a really special girl.

She is in a much better place, heaven, as heaven is a great place (I have touched it), it is full of unconditional love, light and freedom, freedom to just be. I know she is happier there, however it is who she leaves behind who feel they are suffering and for sure they are, suffering a big loss, for this girl and her mom were best friends, they leaned on each other in life. She will be dearly missed by my aunt and uncle as their hearts break for not being in her physical company anymore and sharing all those hugs and I love you's. I was lucky I just saw her and her family last October, me and my mom made a road trip to see them as we felt we had to. My cousin was so very surprised and happy to see us (we surprised them). It was fun and I am glad, she and we, had that time while she was here in the physical world to giggle a bit and share hugs and I love yous. (she deeply appreciated her family)

My heart breaks and aches for my aunt tho as I am unsure how she will process this, you must, as I say earlier in the book, feel, deal and heal. It is certainly a process and takes time.

I don't understand when people pass that people sometimes get excluded as such. In weddings sure, I understand because often there is a cost associated with it and a "guest list" of sorts. But a funeral, it should be open doors to anyone who their life touched in any way. It helps us all feel, deal and heal. I shall be there for when my aunt and uncle need me and want to talk. Me and my aunt are close. I will have to rely on the good times recently shared and just say prayers that she is safe with god and happy.

My dear cousin was a true light and love while here and even tho 35 years is shortlived, she made it seem like she was here for 80 years the way she touched people and was so inclusive of everyone. She was a sensitive girl, as me and may aunt are and she was adopted, so really wanted in my aunts life. She was loved unconditionally and forever will be remembered.

So whatever it takes to grieve you must find a way as you cannot hang onto grief, you have to eventually let go and you will know that time, no one else can tell you. Just feel, remember the good times, deal, deal with the loss, and heal , heal the ache for missing their hugs in life. Try to live as they would and be happy and follow their example of who they were and how they treated others, that is how you can best honour someone and never focus on the negative as we are all so prone to naturally do, only dwell in the positive of things as that is where we should bask.

Being positive brings hope and optimism and joy into ones life and we reflect this and share this energy with others, impacting to a degree their life, so be wise about what energy you give others. It is important for people to come together at such a time too but if unable to, then praying works too and using the phone or email to tell them you are always present for them when they need, that brings people together no matter the miles.

This life is about loss unfortunately, having and then letting go. It is thusly said then that we should appreciate all we are given for the time we have them. That is it, it is just that simple, then we do not live in regret. Always do your best with people and in including others, esp the less advantaged who suffer greatly and often in silence as did my cousin. She felt so much pain but offered to others her joy for life, this was her gift, to not dwell on the negative or pass it around like a ball. I have learned a great deal from her and happy I can dedicate this section to her in my first book. I feel very much for people who suffer from disabilities in life as people are so very hard on one another and not accepting, they have unfound fears mostly and lack compassion.

My cousin was an old soul for sure and will now be an angel in the skies for us all. I hope she looks over us all through these troubling and hard times on earth as we all learn our lessons and live our journeys. It is angels who offer unconditional love, see all and help everyone. She and my aunt believed in angels. Angels are our guiding lights and we should try to tune into them and their guidance when and if we can, as we plug along. Be safe in the knowledge there is a place such as heaven and we all get there eventually, such a place of beauty and peace, no strife.

We are all here to help alleviate pain and suffering of others.

Beware **takasubo syndrome** ("broken heart syndrome"): Takasubo Syndrome is also called Broken Heart Syndrome. One should be aware of it and it affects those left behind by a loss of another. The heart can be so affected by sadness and grief that is becomes deformed and lacks the proper functioning and pumping ability. It becomes mishapen. Sometimes, when one spouse dies, the other will soon follow within 6 months- 1 year due to this. One can also lose their life this way over a child too I believe, if so grief stricken. It may be worth investigating or asking your doctor about this if you find you don't feel well, are weak, fatigued, poor appetite and very grief stricken over a loss of a loved one. It is quite easy to avoid just by being aware it can happen.

God bless you my lovely cousin and rest well 'our sweet angel'

her motto to live by :

> Live in the light, not the shadows…..breath light into others. always say "I love you".

GOD WILL LIGHT THE WAY…..(random thoughts)

cast aside fear and doubt, don't worry worry can make you age and sick.
don't let people disvalue you- ignore it, they live in darkness, in the shadows.
you don't need anyones approval in life but gods and doing what is right in your heart.

"it takes time to feel"

just stepping stones, nothing bad happens to us, just challenges to push us to grow as otherwise we would not, nor reach our true potential.
trust we are always headed in the right direction or maybe there will be a u-turn.
we are in valleys to climb higher mountains but doesn't mean we need to dwell or focus on being in these valleys. everything is temporary, both greatness and weakness .

there is nothing more exciting in life than discovering your true purpose, whether that be driving a truck, serving food, cooking, or writing a book.

believe and have faith in god, good will come along, you will meet the right people in your life, you will achieve abundance in your heart.

share , give of yourself and remain humble, for you were once a student too.
we are all students of life.

let people lead and you follow, know also when to lead and let them follow.

we all have a purpose, no matter how small or insignificant it may seem at the time, it is our phase, our cycle.

I was once a student and didn't "get it" now I feel I can be a leader and a teacher as I have learned so much thru my struggles and triumphs over them.

be inspired and inspire.

don't give into pain and lean on crutches, see it thru to the end and it is in the end where you will triumph. Remain hopeful, positive and optimistic always.
have trust and faith that things are as they should be and be patient with people and mostly yourself. Patience is a true art.

thinking is a skill we take for granted, we can train ourselves to think positive or negative, depending on our habits and direction. Use powerful thoughts, to turn how you feel about something, around.

feed your body good food, your mind good thoughts and your spirit good energy. For then you we be fulfilled and live to your potential. They should be all in balance and have strength for you to be strong and persevere.

we are here for how ever long we don't know, just always remember to just try your best and live true to your heart, if you are determined and a fighter then fight for what is right, if you sit by the side lines and are support then so do that. everyone has a role to play.

we are not responsible for our reputation, try to let that notion go, you will be happier. The truth always gets revealed anyway, one way or another.
don't dwell in someone else's misery, let them be alone if you are not friends........"don't let the bastards grind you down"

we should spend words as we do money, not foolishly.
people we meet hold the keys to our locked doors,
and may help us open them, leading to more enlightenment.

"Sometimes it takes seeing ugly before we can truly appreciate beautiful"

FEAR, ANGER & SELF- PITY

Fear has two brothers, self doubt and anger. So try not to live in fear, for you will be miserable. I only have one thing to say about anger and that is 'He who angers only hurts himself'. It is an utter waste of time, energy and health to be or remain angry. Especially with family. We all have to learn forgiveness and have compassion for people making mistakes. For all of us are only human, and flawed. I know people who waste their energy and thoughts and duly health over being angry at others. They are very sick in the mind and in the body. It is literally killing them, so that if this is your preference of how to die and essentially how you wish to live so be it, but there are definitely healthier ways to deal with people making mistakes. One of these is being proactive, start a charity, change a law, make a law, but your energy into something productive, helpful and positive. Help society don't hinder it.

Anger and self-pity are very interrelated. One almost always relies on the other to exist. Self-pity I will cover in little more detail here. Self-pity is when someone says or thinks "poor me"– a Victim mentality. Often someone has hurt them or they made bad choices in life. They're full of guilt, regret, anger and loneliness. They just think negative all the time about themselves and others. When we indulge in self pity we often feel alone and helpless, not empowered at all.

The only way to get out of self-pity is to change your thinking patterns, literally your thoughts. And with this will come a change in attitude. Mainly one has to let go of the past and live in the moment and be optimistic about the future. Sometimes depression can often get one into a cycle of self-pity. This can often become a vicious and lonely cycle. No one wants to be around someone who self-pity's. No one. So if you wish to be around inspiring people, you yourself must become inspiring. We get what we give.

Often people who self-pity don't realize they are, they're so deep in it. It must either be reflected upon and realized or often is helpful if pointed out by a close friend. Starting point to change is awareness, step one. Then getting a plan is step two. Then step three is putting the plan into action and creating good habits both mental and physical. Step four is making it a habit.

You must take a stand and love yourself, love everything about you, flaws and all, triumphs and disappointments. For there is no failure in trying in life, only in not trying. We regret what we don't do, not what we do. Humans have great hindsight so we see problems more easily after-the-fact, thus we are harder on ourselves and others for mistakes.

"You can't feel anger and be thankful at the same time"

"Anger always hurts just one person, and that is the one who feels it"

So step one: Awareness

Becoming self-aware can be so hard, -to look in the mirror.... often what bothers us in others is because we are looking in the mirror, so realize your thinking patterns. Be honest with yourself.
Ask yourself often, how do I see me, others and the world. Reflect.

Step two: Plan

Make a plan. Set out how you are going to practice thinking positive and change emotional patterns, whether thru meditation, caring for others, volunteering. Stop comparing. Write out this plan if you must and follow it. Stop the negative patterns and turn positive.

Step three: Putting the plan into Action

Put into action your plan– with Discipline, steady and consistent. Keep a calendar or journal if you can. Reflect on your progress. Check- in.

Step four: Making it a habit

Make sure you develop healthy habits. Catch yourself thinking negative and turn it around. Within about three weeks to three months you will notice your behaviour become habit and eventually after about one year your life will change and you will feel differently, people will like to be around you and you will enjoy life. You'll become a thankful person instead of bitter. This will then help dissipate any anger as you can't be angry and thankful at the same time. If you do find you have bad habits, generally you cannot rid yourself of them but rather you replace them. Be conscious you are replacing bad habits with good habits. Try to live a healthier happier life, for you and others around you. Again never self-pity, is a deep dark hole that is hard to see and if unaware, not able to get out of. Become a Victor, instead of this victim you've created.

ACCEPT DIFFERENT

We all like the same things, like sheep, we all think if others are indulging it must be right. Wrong. To be different than the rest is to be strong, march to the beat of your own drum, have the self confidence in all your decisions. Stand out. This is all very challenging as people are drawn to what makes them feel comfortable (most are) as they often will choose a mate who resembles them, even pets sometimes, we all like to hang out with people who look like we do, act like we do and think like we do. You see it all the time in cliques. I hate to say it but people are essentially sheep. It takes real guts to just be who you truly are and not care about any judgement or lack of acceptance. It works that we are sheep because deep down we all just want to be accepted, a part of the group , to be included and essentially liked. This feeds our self esteem and makes us feel strong and powerful as we often look outwards for acceptance and the world around us to do this for us.

But really we must look inward, accept ourselves, realize who we really are, what we truly like and dislike, our values and our own passions, Become an individual. In this sense we should all encourage people to be different and for it is when people are different and become friends and spend time together that they truly learn from each other and dissipate their innate judgement tendency. It builds compassion and understanding. We are not to feel separate from others just because they may dress different, look different or behave different (maybe not as smart). We must practice patience and see every person in our lives as an opportunity to grow, spiritually , for that is why we exist, to grow on our paths and journey.

It is very hard not to be accepted I will agree and most people feel very out of sorts in a crowd they find little acceptance in. However, you must remain strong in who you are, have faith in who you are and how you present and try to teach those around you, no matter how slowly it happens, your value as an individual, some may come around, some not, it will bring the cream to the top so to say and you will find these that accept you under all conditions will be quality people and your best friends you can count on, the rest would be considered phoney and interested in their own purposes.

So step out, step up, be who you are and above all remain brave and faithful in it, express who you are and the more people who indulge in being different the more people will become accustomed to seeing this and accepting it and accepting you, if you care whether they do or not. Most importantly accept yourself, unconditionally, love those special parts of yourself, like being like no other, an original, unique, celebrate it at every opportunity. Be you as only you can be.

I am an artist and my work is so different for where I live and is hardly accepted (they like soft colors here), I don't care at all, I love it and have fun and one day I know it will be accepted, maybe when I am gone, like some artists, but for the moment I don't care, I accept and enjoy it, and to me that is the number one key to life, do what you love and keep going. Often too I dress differently and act a little eccentric so am not accepted this way, (I march to the beat of my own drum), I can be overly friendly which makes some uncomfortable as most are used to being professional or cold. I am open, unique, strong, brave, determined and live my passions and that is more important to me than being accepted into a crowd I may come to not appreciate later on. For in the end we all must only live with ourselves and in a forever changing world the only thing that doesn't change is our uniqueness and spirit, ...So celebrate and encourage it. Don't hide it.

Get to know who you are and express it with gratitude and fortitude.

Also Challenge yourself and start becoming friendly with those that are different than you, you will learn alot.

LIVE IN THE LIGHT NOT THE DARK

We can choose to live in love (light) or we can live in fear (dark). Don't fear anymore, have trust, hope, no anger, move forward, don't stay stuck.

Fear has sisters and cousins, they are 'worry", "anger", vengeance", "ego", hate, regret, hurt, addictions.
Love is freedom, to feel joy, and peace and glory and hope, open heart and mind, you think better and are more creative.

How to live in light:
We can decide to step into the light vs. live in darkness, in the fear. And to do this we must, when we decide to live in the light, take our first few steps in the light not in darkness. Let go of fear- how ?- change your mind about how you approach things , how you want to live. Start a good habit of thinking, Say Ok I feel the fear, let it move through you and let it go as just a thought and feeling. Don't stay there in it. Then turn your thoughts back to good. Relax, sit back, say OK I feel fed, take a deep breath, feel it, let it move thru you and out of you, take another deep breath of relief it is gone and get your mind back to positive and joy and no fear. Like a shock we let go of.

Choice:
Make a choice, a conscious one that will later turn to subconscious of how you wish to think, live and affect others. We cannot hang onto darkness, fear and the devil. We must learn to let go and in a sense ignore little stuff. We do have a choice in what we think and thusly how we feel. Only you are responsible for this too, not others.

Healthy Mind living in the light:

Mental illness and strife can come from the stress of negative and fear based thinking- hurts, injures the mind. Just like stress can affect heart attacks, negative and stressful fear based thinking can affect the health of the mind, even to the point of a mental breakdown or depression (I like to call it a "mind attack").

When we live in the light, we feel joy and peace and this becomes less a strain on the mind, depression can subside, you feel less anxious and delusions and paranoia may even be kept at bay. Whatever the mental illness, it is healthy for the mind especially to live in the light and feel peace and ease. Work hard and move forward into the positive things in your life, don't be held back by the heavy, the things that weigh you, don't , especially negatively. Make better choices. Move slowly out of the frame of mind of fear and take chances on the good. When you see a fork in the road to go right or left, choose the path of least resistance.

Lessons from your past:

It is ok to take our lessons of times of struggle and darkness in to the future as reminders of what we learned and of how far we have come. It is impossible sometimes to just forget. So take it with you like you would a tool into the positive future, only as a reminder, not a way to think or live or remain stuck. It will help strengthen you into the future to remember what your times of struggle taught you. As it is only in our times of challenges where we grow and strengthen our character, become who we were meant to be. So look at lessons of the past as good things and future tools.

We must learn to rejoice during our trials:

Be happy and rejoice during your times of trial and supposedly "suffering" for it means you will grow and are growing, either building compassion and empathy, learning valuable lessons and wisdom or able to assist others going thru the 'same' sometime down the road. It doesn't serve to feel stuck and get negative during these times, for you should be wide open to whatever and whoever enters your life to help you. These people are important as they will help you reach beyond your trial(s) and eventually come out of it, as a more humane and wiser being. When you "get" this earned wisdom, "guard it" and then try to "practice it" often. Protect it as you would a precious belonging.

Trials often bring out more our talents, our courage and confidence. This is the exciting part! Trials can make us stronger, tougher, more wise OR they can defeat us, only you decide. It is when we rejoice during our trials and meet them head on that it is usually a favourable outcome. Remember, get wise, protect your wisdom and grow your wisdom (use it). Wisdom cannot be purchased with money. It can only be gained by experience or sometimes extreme paying attention.

Destiny:

Be helpful to others, don't feel like you need to teach anyone a lesson or get back at them.. Simply let it move thru you the hurt one may have caused you, Feel, heal and deal…then move on. Let it go by, like you would a racing car that almost hit you. Don't let that sensation linger, the fear and hate. Don't stay scared. No one can hold you back or keep you from your destiny except you. When you let others control your behaviour, you make wrong decisions for yourself and it causes strife, suffering and more pain in your life.

Opportunity/ benefits :

Essentially darkness is where satan resides, ….light is god- good and hope. Don't get drawn into darkness. We never know how long we have to live, so why spend so much time in darkness, what a waste. To live in the light and spend time there you will feel love and joy, two emotions that help feed the soul and give us reason to live. By being easy on the mind too, your physical will benefit- be more healthy, and pain free, less suffering. For we are not really here to suffer but to live. It is when we get stuck in this

trap of fear based thinking we experience suffering and hurt, needlessly. If one lives in dark , they live in frustration and debt. When you decide to live in the light, at least move towards it, god will present new, better options, put them right in front of you. Good opportunities will present themselves. Choose them.
When we live in the light , it is a place of forgiveness and compassion for people and their mistakes.

When we live in fear and anger this draws negative energy towards us (otherwise known as murphys law!) and we begin to then experience more of the same and get even more stuck in this pattern and misery. However, when we learn to live in love and forgiveness we draw the positive in life towards us creating great opportunity and growth and being prosperous and happy.
It is kinda like the "like attracts like" theory, real simple when you think about it and live it.

"The only one holding you back is YOU"

TRUTH

You know "truth" is a funny thing. Often we can never get it even from ourselves. Realistically the only place we could really find truth is within ourselves when we look deep and honestly. Most people don't do this though, they have reasons for hiding the truth whether insecurities, self-deception or plain denial. Why is it so hard for people to tell others the truth. All I look for in friendship is an honest one, a place and relationship where we can tell each other exactly how we feel and think about ourselves and the other person and situations. This is so very hard in most relationships though because people have many reasons for hiding the truth from others whether it be their own ego, their being manipulative, scared, insecure or fear losing the relationship. It is difficult for famous people when they're surrounded by yes-men, these people will never tell them the truth, only agree with them and foster their bad habits and foster bad thoughts and always have their motivation of not wanting to lose the relationship because especially possibly they're being paid by these people. This is the most dangerous thing to happen to famous people is to surround themselves and their Inner circle with people who won't tell them the truth. If they don't have these people who tell them the truth they can easily go down the rabbit hole, often on their own and it is a difficult struggle back. Most of the time this rabbit hole becomes addictions and often drugs. These people who are yes-men in fact act as crutches and enablers to this person's actions and in response to them.

Is a very special thing to surround yourself with an inner circle who will be honest, up front and secure with you and the relationship. Realistically, A relationship that is not honest Will never be filled with trust and will be fruitless and useless in the end, simply just an exercise of deception. Some people value friendships no matter how empty, fragile or fake they may actually be. These are the type of relationships I do not value, for it is hard to get my trust and harder to lose but once you've lost it, it is extremely difficult to get back if ever possible. I'm extremely loyal to my friends, I am direct and I am honest with them and I try to be honest with who I am. I believe relationships should be give-and-take, each person taking time listening to the other and each person doing the talking. A real relationship takes the shape of people trying to get to know each other and help each other in their journey. We all need friends but what we need to learn to value is those honest and sincere ones. Even if the relationship gets put in jeopardy and is lost because of honesty, it is lost for a good reason and at least these two people can live honest lives, even if separate. I am quite unique in that I am direct, Assertive, as honest as I can be and I will tell you what I think based on my experience in life, my knowledge, my intelligence, intuition and how I can support you. I will not support someone if I think they're being extremely crazy and not thinking correctly, I will rather tell them that I think this based on who I am, which could include some inexperience towards this other person and their situation so therefore I should not judge so much but rather go along with them if they can find the truth in their craziness. It is a true friend who will tell you you're crazy when you are being crazy. There's nothing wrong with this as we all get crazy sometimes as it turns out some of the best ideas in the world seems like the craziest. I get crazy ideas all the time, with reality being that it is sometimes these crazy ideas I get that cease to surprise me, as life is full of surprises and I really put nothing past people and what they're capable of. (sometimes you can support crazy)

 Deception is on the rise in life as we're losing that true honesty and sincerity in relationships, that trust and tightness that should exist and we all rely on the Internet for our communication nowadays by texting and losing our thoroughness. People don't have time to be thorough anymore, they just go along with things saying yes, yes I'm busy, I'll get back to you on that, etc. Relationships take time, people just don't have this nor value this anymore, they're so busy doing such inconsequential Little things surrounding them in life that they can't focus on the big stuff, is like that saying you can't see the forest for the trees …..everybody's busy focusing on the trees instead of the forest that they are in. Communication has changed.

Our privacy is another thing, we lost this and it is so easy for people to know whatever they like about another person without going through them but rather they go through Mr. Google. Mostly everyone has a footprint called an Internet footprint on the web and for all to see, at any time. It is a mistake that we trust this Internet and that we are so loose and relaxed about putting information, pictures and our most valued thoughts On this thing called the web. It all goes on there unscrutinized but later to be scrutinized closely. The web can put an end to many relationships and help not even begin them. It interferes and it should cause us much worry. As we should treat the Internet as, if it's something you can't tell your mother, then don't put it on the Internet, it also goes if you can't show it to your mother, don't put it on the Internet. We lack true, honest, thorough and upfront Communication, everybody hides behind the Internet in being who they are and it fosters deception and that we can hide behind a computer and almost say anything we want, thinking nobody will ever know the truth. Often this happens and people get taken advantage of especially by the bad people where they hide within the Internet. At times the truth does get finally revealed and people do get caught but this happens less rather than more. I fear for society and that everyone secludes themselves in their own little bubble and will be so disconnected, everybody will be fighting for their own survival instead of leaning on each other for help, support and honesty. It will become a disgruntled and disjointed society where the weak will get weaker, the poor will get poorer and the rich probably richer but more lonely.

The Internet, while a useful tool, has helped foster a true loneliness that people feel. A real disconnect from the community and especially their closest friends. Facebook works as an interface between friends but it is all quite fake as you can never really know the truth unless you see a person, feel a person and really hear the person. We're losing that human touch, A true intimacy between human beings and sharing. We often, now more than ever turn to our pets for this unconditional love as we must find it somewhere and this is why people go so nuts in how they treat their pets in that people treat them like a fellow human being when they are in fact simply a simple animal. In Pets at least people can value that they do receive the unconditional love and it comforts them and helps ease them in their loneliness.

Truly though we must come back to a place where we share, care and foster each other's feelings, insecurities, struggles and suffering. We must assist each other on our individual journeys without judgment but with the best honesty we could possibly have. Loyalty and trust really don't exist anymore in relationships. This is very sad as that is the basis of relationships, if they are not built on loyalty and trust, they are fake and empty. We will simply live in a fantasy world, full of deception and fakeness where everybody acts just like on TV as everyone tries to be like and model the people they see in the media. Our relationship with media is growing ever more intense as people are hooked on their iPhones, Facebook, Twitter and now Netflix, it seems we just can't get enough of this technology as it feeds us thoughts and drives our inspiration and passions which can be fleeting. I think as technology is wonderful, it has it's place as a tool that is overused and believed in and we depend upon that it so much it becomes a dangerous zone, that if it ever fails us we feel nothing but frustration and lost.... no reality to ground us or people in our lives who will really be there for us when we need them. The down side (as there is one to every situation) is the Internet is really dangerous as it holds so much power and control and invades our privacy to such an extreme degree that anyone can have our private passwords that we value and sometimes we make so simple. It seems there are passwords for everything nowadays and it gets confusing so people will simplify their passwords and end up being hacked and their privacy gone.

The Internet helps foster paranoia as nobody is ever sure if their e-mail or the computer are ever being looked at and computers record our every fingerprint and everything we look at in its hardware which is saved forever within the computer until it is erased. Very few people erase their computers, is like their past can easily catch up with them at the push of a button. Nothing we ever do anymore has privacy attached to it. This is dearly connected to honesty in that if we feel our privacy is always on parade we will be less honest with ourselves and others. Technology has certainly raised our anxiety levels in life.

I have a friend who always speaks of truth, that in life, that we must find the truth and I live for the truth myself. I believe the truth always prevails and will always be known in the hearts of the people involved. Karma comes into play in that people know what they do to each other and how they lie and in the end they just live with themselves even if there is nothing called justice. Justice has also failed us deeply in turn as people with all their money, technology, ways to manipulate and deceive and all their lies can beat a person who only has truth to stand on but because they have no money, have difficulty in proving it. Is often an unfair fight nowadays where the rich win and often they can buy their way out of jail but the poor remain in jail as they don't have the money to either buy people or the technology or knowledge to help them fight and get out. It is true some honest people and good people exist in our jails as they are innocent and mistakes been made in putting them there. But for the most part people who have been caught in wrongdoings do spend time in jail and for some it is not enough time. It is truly an unfair justice system nowadays that we cannot rely upon, it is so twisted and unsupportive to the truth and really again all about who has the most money and power.(generally speaking of course) For sometimes it is those people who have money and/or hold political positions especially, who can be deceptive towards the public and get away with it when they actually belong in jail for what they do and say.

Do I believe in justice? I am not sure of this question because I still am naïve and enVision the truth as prevailing even though the wheels of justice turn ever so slowly and may not favour the truth. Therefore as I come back to truth it is really only the truth within and about ourselves that we can ever really know, depend on and live by. An honest life lived is a good one and one to be proud of.

So don't try to expect to find the truth from the exterior, from others, from the environment or even what we strive to do in life, Look within yourself and reflect as often as you can about where you're at and how you can live a more honest life with those you care about and try to be as honest as you can with them, for this fosters respect and self-respect. We are not here to waste each other's time with lies but to cherish and value time and treat people with respect they deserve in telling them the truth whether you think they can bear to hear it or not. How people receive the truth is not your responsibility but rather theirs, you just have to know your purpose and intent in telling them the truth and hopefully it is always to help them, and not hurt them like out-of-spite, say during a battle. Is important that you know your intent and so does this other person, so that they don't not become defensive but rather open and receptive. Intent is a tricky thing to know because it really involves the truth. Often when we get angry we blurt out our truths whether they be right or wrong. Our filter and thusly guard, is virtually on vacation when we blow our top. I don't know how it is, but it is then that we speak our minds, tho angry is not well received and puts the other person on the defensive.

In conclusion I again state that we can only rely on the truth within ourselves and live the truth outwardly from within. We must share the truth with all we are close to, those at work, those in the community, our friends and our family and try to live an honest, upright, respectful Life. The truth can be contagious actually and you'll find when you open up to somebody and be honest they might react in opening up to you and being honest in return almost like a smile, something sincere and with good intent it Will likely be returned with the same attitude. So try to live an honest life mostly towards yourself and certainly don't expect to find honesty and the truth from outside yourself, at least so readily. I once told a friend that I would rather watch peoples actions and how they behave than the words that come out of their mouth as the words can often be twisted, manipulative and dishonest. The body speaks the truth in that it is a subconscious reaction that we don't realize is taking place but body language is so very important, and as honest as you will see and get from people. So try to study how people behave, how they act and how they respond with their body if you wish to know the truth and take their words with a grain of salt, depending on the level of your relationship.

Never feel insulted by anybody's words as often these words can be empty and wrong. Very few people in this world Will truly get to know you on a level where what comes out of their mouth towards you Will be the truth. So try not to let words ever hurt you even though they hold that power to. We are unique creatures as we have speech in that it forms words and language but then there animals such as whales who have a language of themselves with sounds, and really words are sounds strung together. The difference being between us and animals, is animals have a better ability to be honest in their communication and sounds towards each other without the intent of the ego getting in the way, it's vindictiveness or manipulative ability. It is a joy to watch other creatures communicate using sound especially the way we hear birds and other animals, it reminds us that there really are truly honest ways to communicate.

DON'T TAKE OFFENCE

This portion of the book is about not taking offence to how people behave towards you or what they may say. It is easy for us as sensitive human beings to take offence easily and hold people and their opinions in higher regard than ourselves. But we must protect our hearts, Guard them, put up walls around them to protect them from this negativity and offence from others. This is a process of being aware of people's intent when they talk to you and give you their opinion or if they treat you badly. Joel Osteen has said there will be 25% people who don't like you and never will like you, 25% of people who won't like you but Could like you, 25% would like you but can eventually not like you, And 25% of people who will JUST like you. These are good ratios and makes a lot of sense, this is easy to keep in mind when you are aware of it when you're trying to please that 25% who will never like you. For pleasing that 25% that will never like you is just a waste of valuable energy. We only have so much energy in our lives and we have to be careful where we spend it and the activities and problems we give it. For we cannot come to the end of our lives and say why did I waste so much time worrying, fretting or being offended by that person or those people. When someone hurts you with words or actions, just think to yourself, will I even recall their name in 5 years, even 1 yr?

Live your life as though your heart is in a vault guarded under lock and key or an army, only let those people in who are deserving and give them your time and energy for those are the people who will assist you in life and support you in all you do and let you live your light. Keep the others out and away and just ignore them.

Often people who have favour upon them too find much opposition in life due mostly to people seeing 'us' and being insecure and jealous and therefore wanting to put us down. They "see" easily your favour and your gifts and want to somehow bring you down to their level where they exist. Insecurity is against these people who don't support you but you must guard your heart against them and not let them in. If you do let them in they will only waste your time and energy and frustrate you because that 25% is never going to favour or like you, no matter what you do or how kind you are to them. In letting in this 25%, it will only help defeat your confidence and make you feel horrible and give you nothing but worry and low self-esteem. Try to focus instead on the 25% that like you and live your life knowing that those middle 25% others can switch to "liking you" or "not liking you" and that is mostly up to them not you. Live your life and spend your energy as though you would money, enjoy yourself, Live life to your fullest and don't let "energy vampires" suck you dry and keep you from your dreams. It takes time to build up these walls and realize who's against you and who is for you but go by your gut instincts and signs, physical signs as 'actions' speak louder than words. If you want to give someone a small chance do, but don't give them too much of yourself in this process.

We must always protect our hearts as it is the most precious thing about us and stress does us no good, only positive stress which may come from living our dreams and being supported by those positive people around us. Stress, worry, fret, frustration and feeling down on yourself and question yourself and having little confidence is not good for your health at all and will eventually cause your physical systems to break down as your mental is greatly affected. So protect your mental and physical at all times and try to live as full and long life as you possibly can (with quality), it is hard to ignore these people who cause you grief but try your best and just walk away, learn to let it go, let them go and try to remove yourself from bad situations and those people. They will be frustrated as you walk away as you have become a target and they enjoy bringing you down (their ego) but thus eventually they will move on to new targets to be jealous about.

People can become easily offended, don't be one of those, as I say don't waste your energy or time and block these people and their comments out of your mind. Try not to engage in details, stories and gossip about others or negative situations. Make it your goal in life not to be offended and how you do this is by "forgiving others", not judging them and not holding them in higher regard than yourself. You can give people respect but at the same time don't hold them higher than yourself nor their opinions. As only you can really know who you are and what you're capable of and where you're headed and most importantly where you've been and the lessons you've learned. It is very difficult when we work with these people and they become bullies and harassers and we must stay engaged as we cannot walk away so easily. There is the option to quit and move on if you're not too attached to the job or there are other opportunities, to save your heart and soul from this person's bullying and demeaning you and in the end wasting your energy and just giving you hurt.

But if you cannot quit, you must meet this person head on and stand up to them and let the chips fall where they may, hopefully with a superior in the room at the time as a witness so you are not further sabotaged at your place of work. You must see it as not your problem but their problem they're miserable, they feel insecure and they feel threatened or intimidated by you, this feeling of theirs may never go away no matter what you say or do or how you try to help them. These people simply are who they are and they never change or they never learned their lessons or try to be helpful human beings. ... I often categorize people as being helpful or hurtful. You know which group you want to be around and who will nurture you on your path and journey. Try to avoid the hurtful ones at all costs and give them none of your time or energy, what you can do is live is an example for them to follow but not engage with them. This is the best you can do towards a hurtful person. Have compassion actually for them and almost feel sorry for them as it is true what goes around comes around in a sense of Karma and they will get hit by the hurt they send around. Knowing this reality will help you deal with them on a better level with patience, tolerance and compassion, in a sense making you better and more of who you are. Try to use them to your advantage in the sense of growing these attributes of patience, tolerance and compassion which are tough to attain in life and often practice.

In conclusion always protect and guard your heart especially from harmful poisons and don't let people eat up your time and energy, for it is valuable, one of the most valuable things you have even over money. You would let somebody Rob you of your money ?.... so don't let anyone rob you of your energy either. Build these walls and let only the special people in your life, that special 25% and possibly a few others who will and can support you and ignore the others as best you can. Don't always be so open and an easy target for these villains out there. Try never to take offence, as hard as this is you must practice it and keep it at the forefront of your mind.

And again mostly the secret to this is to have a forgiving heart and to easily let go, especially of hurtful comments and putdowns. Another is to see these people as smaller beings then yourself, don't give them much attention or regard. Consider the source. They may be less evolved then you, less favoured.

CREATE LOVE

(dedicated to my good friend Andrew who taught me) 10/24/14

Grieving, is it narcissistic & self pity or a feeling of loss? Is this the same thing?
I always believed it was pure self - pity like one of my friends says, to grieve, especially a long time. However I rather now feel it is quite natural to grieve, we feel a loss, an emptiness and it feels like an open wound, then we go thru it and heal and realize we can go on and be ok. This takes time and process.
It is cold to feel that it is all self involved and self pity as our heart goes out to families, those left behind and left with a loss of support and love from this person. One of my friends said to me "how can you grieve and your heart go out at the same time"?..., easy I say you can feel loss for others, an empathy and compassion. You feel sorry. Feeling sorry is valid and expresses you are not a cold human being or psychopath. This is always a good sign. How long do we grieve for though, this is important, as if long it can wear on our health and hurt us, leaving us worse off than before the person departed. It helps to express and talk about it as we all need this, a shoulder to lean on and share our experiences, happy or sad with. So go ahead and grieve, it is natural and healthy and means you are alive.

(Some people lie and hurt others in order to "get even"…..)
How do we grieve tho when people hurt us or lie and get away with it? This I will discuss in detail as I have lately experienced people betraying me and lying in court and it going against me in every way. How do people live with themselves or get away with this? Well I have learned above all this is just reality, people hurt each other and look out for their own best interests, call it narcissism as it is certainly on the rise with money becoming our new god. People will step on you with power and money and putdowns if they are up against the wall and get caught doing something they don't take responsibility for.

What do we do in response to people hurting us or lying?…we try to "Create Love". Create love instead of helping create more problems from these folks. No one can stop you from living your dreams if you wish to move forward with your talents. I use to try to " set people straight on the truth" and this only got me deeper in trouble and a big headache, affecting my health too. It is discouraging to know that people can lie and actually get away with it, especially if they have power and money. I use to have a great deal of respect for this doctor and his wife and they were both church people, wow did they shock me recently, lying Under Oath, about something where there was evidence, although not real clear, it existed and still they deny everything.

How can this happen? Oh how it hurts when people you least expect to do this, do. An enemy you'd expect, but church people and a doctor to boot doing this ? Hard to believe. It hurts and one way to deal with this pain is take it and create love with it, don't let them win. Often it is money motivated and people trying to protect their own reputations while they destroy yours. They simply don't care about you. Sad but true, it happens and expect it when you least expect it.

How do I create love ?....I draw, paint, meditate, journal, write, spread hope and optimism and try to care about/help others. This emits a positive feeling which can often defeat any negative that exists and will often stop the enemy in their tracks as they realize they did not get the best of you.

Life is too short, don't focus on those who hurt and lie rather put your energy into how you can make this place a better place to be even if only for one person. You have to examine, if I had two weeks to live, what would I do with my time, fight? I doubt it, rather you would try to live. So keep this in mind, live, don't indulge people in fighting and don't really fight for the truth when it hurts you, rather know that these people who lie have to live with themselves and believe in Karma which exists. It catches up with people eventually in their own lessons.

People get humbled by their own life experiences and this draws certain people into their lives, people who will mean something to them. So don't begrudge your experiences or trials, rather take them in and learn from them and be humble, not arrogant for we all have problems, all of us. Some problems never even get resolved, with some don't try. If you cannot resolve, try to change, don't complain about it, you empower it then. Give praise always to those who listen and support you in your dreams and your experiences and even sadness.

Praise does a lot more then complaining, complaining spreads negativity and negativity is draining, praise is positive energy and invigorates us. Never take anyone for granted. Part of our grieving (to get back to that), is when we never had a chance to say goodbye and say thank you to those who touch our lives and believe in us. This fills in your heart as deep regret, why didn't I …..why….. shoot….now I won't ever have the chance, but don't believe this, you can still say things and they hear us, give them thanks even when they depart, say it out loud, tell friends about how these departed touched your life and what they meant, boast about them, they will surely hear this and appreciate it and it will fill your heart with joy, displacing grief. Eventually you will feel good again and meet new people who will help you out as well. There are good people out there, don't let the small few dirty people drag you down and under. Don't get caught in their lies and cycle of hatred. Never.

SIMILAR CIRCUMSTANCES ,TWO COMPLETELY DIFFERENT OUTCOMES

When we pity ourselves we begin to take on the visual appearance that others should pity us as well. All we do then is learn to complain about our challenge(s) or circumstance(s). This does no one any good and is very unproductive for society as a whole. Don't complain, do something about it.

It's 4 am and I am writing this book here , I be at emergency at VGH with suspected food poisoning from couple days ago, not cleared up yet. I am waiting while working on my book to finish it once and for all. (this is my last blurb) This guy sits down across from me with a pole, slightly younger and talks to me. Says "what are you doing, gee your computer is thin". I replied "Yes I'm a writer and carry it around with me to write". He asked what are you writing about, I said "fibromyalgia", he then replied "oh that, that is all in your head" (as he points to his head). I said no it is very physical, your mental is tied to your physical, the brain is physically broken. I Mentioned "I like writing , you here might just make it into my book too". I added, "it has taken me 4 years to write it and all I wish is to help just one person recover and be healthy again".

Now here is a guy who looks real unhealthy, tells me how he has Crohns disease, had since 9 y/o, no cure for ,blah, blah, blah ...complaining how hard his life is, how he has NO ONE, on disability, on narcotics (opiates and the such). He looked thin, unshaven, straggly, sick, didn't care, wanted pity and attention. He wanted to tell someone his aches. (I listened and was compassionate, trying my best not to judge but rather inspire). He was apparently waiting for them to ready a room upstairs as he had a flare- up of Crohns (infection). Now I don't know much about Crohns but do know it can be very challenging to have, in fact I told him when I get home I am googling it to learn about it.

I said to this guy, him looking at me, do you think maybe I've endured even more than you have, he replied "oh no", I said "I know , I don't wear it". "I am a very determined person to better myself, no matter what and it serves me well". I continued, "hearing your story I have in fact been thru more than you have and have no one too". A cat (plus a few 'angels'). I said "and here I am using what I have to write a book to help others". (there is alot more I've been thru than just fibro !). I said to him (his name is Leo), I said Leo why not write poetry, a book, something, do something before you die, he said "Yah I used to write good poetry", I then replied "good, then do it , will be good for you to use your talents, we all have talents and something to offer this world" " just do it, think positive and put yourself into something positive vs. dwelling on the negative." (I don't know if he listened to me at all but I told him we were probably meant to meet). I told him I watch Joel Osteen sometimes for positive inspiration, he shrugged, not really wanting to follow this advice, I said "just try him out and see if you jive with what he has to say, if you don't just turn it off, no harm". Try it.

World of difference between how he appeared to the world, his attitude and what he was giving compared to me, one who has in many ways endured more, a survivor and feeling no need to feel sorry for myself, nor wear it for the world to see. It's True this plays the disadvantage that I don't appear to need in help when in fact I could use all the help I can get, I still struggle. But I won't wear my woes on my sleeve, I feel too proud to not put my best foot forward.

WE ALL NEED GOLIATHS

We all need Goliaths in life, for without Goliath David would've never become king, He would've always stayed the shepherd boy.You see our Goliaths or rather enemies in life propel us forward, they stir us up, they challenge us to make them wrong and to become all that we can be. Instead of feeling frustrated and hurt by them we should thank our enemies as much as we do our friends as without criticism and negative words against us we would not move forward as quickly or efficiently as otherwise. We would not be spurred on. I have a fellow writer, a Friend, who became a writer because they were faced up against some very prominent and hard testing Lawyers,very strong ones. My friend, in defending their case, they wrote so much in their defence towards their enemies that they sooner or later actually became a writer, a "newfound destiny" in their life. You see God puts enemies in the path of our lives to make us better, to have us be more confident, to challenge us, to believe in ourselves more than anyone else and to be ultimately successful. The next time you have an enemy in your way putting you down don't begrudge them, rather see that they will be a stepping stone for you and promote you, a set up, not a put down, they will after all in the end be of assistance and help you. I know this is hard to understand when you're in the midst of someone being so critical and/or putting you down but you must have the right attitude and hold it dear to your heart that it will ultimately work in your favour, to your advantage not disadvantage, as they so wish. For without difficulties in life we simply do not grow, we won't be able to expand our talents, our confidence, and courage.

We can stay stagnant and stuck when life is always so easy and positive. So next time you see an enemy, take it as an unlikely challenge to become a better you, a more successful you and in the end to make a difference, proving them wrong or that they are actually a fool. Be thankful, content and happy for your enemies, not disgruntled, mad, upset or put off. We all have our lessons and challenges in life and enemies are but just one of these. You will eventually , given time see the good they did for you, not harm, which they may have actually intended.

We all need to belong:
As humans we all have an innate need to belong, to be accepted, whether by someone or into a group. If you find you don't fit, it's probably because it's not meant to be, so Move On, find a place you do fit where you will be more comfortable, where you do belong. I guess we all need to feel this belonging and acceptance, to feel at ease and that we are loved. But sometimes you don't need people to like you or accept you, just as long as you accept yourself and can move along your path in your own Merry way. If you are perceived as "odd" or stand out consider it a compliment as you being an individual, rather than fitting in or at worst trying to fit in. Trying to fit in can expend a lot of energy on your behalf, in the end being a waste of time. For perhaps you actually don't need these others, they perhaps need you more than you need them. You need to find peace

within yourself to move on and move forward, towards the destiny you were chosen for. Nothing happens by accident, for we're all meant to meet the people we meet, learn the lessons we learn and go through the trials we do. To essentially help each other. There is no positive and negative forces, just force. There's a purpose for everything in life and we must pay attention. For when it is that we don't pay attention and we want something that either doesn't belong to us or isn't meant to be we can run into a wall and feel frustrated. Don't waste your energy. Your precious energy. I'm not saying don't try, you could make an effort to do people right but if you find that it doesn't feel right or you can't find a good fit that is when you must move on. Moving on and letting go is really a positive thing in life as is the hardest change or not being accepted. We must accept this letting go and go forward. We will eventually meet the people we were meant to meet and fit in where we're meant to fit in. When you get this, life will be easy and it will feel right and you will feel love.

As I said in the previous part we all need our Goliaths for the push they can give us and to propel us. Critics actually have the ability to make us fight harder. When we just have friends that support us and dote on us we don't tend to grow. We all need a little pressure to succeed and the naysayers, to prove them wrong. Don't worry about it, time will take care of it and these naysayers will be in the end proved wrong. Why people become naysayers or enemies towards others is complicated and can be for so many reasons, most reasons we don't know. Fitting in is not all it's cracked up to be, rather accepting who you are, knowing your integrity, your honesty, your determination and your talents are the most important things in life and that you can give yourself. Don't worry about what others can give or do for you. What you can do for yourself is the most important and prominent focus that you should be focused on. It is foreverlasting to work on yourself, accept yourself and love yourself. For no one can do this for you. It is something you must do for yourself, in the time you were given to do it. It's such a fleeting world nowadays and so easy to go for things that are convenient and easiest and that we think are right for us, but the real place of permanence is how we feel about ourselves, how we treat others and how we live out our destiny. When one dies, all is forgotten about this person except the impact they had on others, their making this world a better place and this is thusly Immortal (lives on). So the next time you see an enemy, take your hand and give them a handshake and a smile, be appreciative rather than sorrowful and feeling pitiful. For it is them who is going to make you more of who you are and stronger, be all your meant to be in this world. Take all friends and enemies in stride, all the good and seemingly bad, accept the times to grow with gumption and walk an admirable path.

Be aware in life that friends can also really be enemies, this phrase coined aptly "frienemies", they don't have your best interests at heart and may be against you (not believe in you). Also be very aware that family can be enemies, a "new" term I have coined (as I have never heard it used before) but the word for these people is "famemy" (or famemies). Watch these wolves in sheeps clothing, who easily fool you, don't let them bring you down or discourage you but rather use them to prop yourself up in life, to strive for greatness beyond anyones expectations. So friends, frienemies, enemies and even famemy, try to embrace them all and use them all to your advantage to step up and step out and become your very best. Always keep this attitude that everyone put in your path is there to help you in some way (they just carry different titles). Just also keep in mind a bus you drive in this thing called life where people hop on and off and sometimes you have to actually "kick" people off your "**bus of life**".

Don't be too shy to do this if they are really a thorn in your side or too abusive towards you. Know what and who you deserve.

A WORD ABOUT FAMILIES

Some family relationships seem or may actually be quite psychotic in nature. You see the relationship is tight and often long, parents see their children thru *every* stage of their life and growth, froma helpless baby to a working adult and children grow up watching their parents. This distorts things immensely for these often precious relationships as a parent can often get stuck in an "image" of their child, no matter what stage and not see them as they are today, developed and changed, grown. And a child can often place too many demands on a parent, expecting unconditional love and support.

The reason I talk about family relationships here is that when one becomes ill within a family, it often strains relationships, as it shifts everyones thinking patterns, expectations and roles of one another. One may become all of a sudden super dependent when they are not used to it, the role shift. It becomes difficult to remove ourselves from old thinking patterns and our images of each other. The main reason these relationships become so strained and psychotic is because either party in the relationship expects too much from the other, whether it be love or support, a hug or money. A parent can place high expectations on their child to perform yet always treat this individual as the student in life as they remain the older one. This can be a strain as when we expect a lot and don't receive it, we become frustrated and disappointed and maybe even tearful over it. Children on the other hand when they become dependent again on their parent due to say illness this can put them back in the scenario of being a needy child, this frightens the parent and frustrates them, challenges their unreal expectations. Too high of expectations on a child can be hard on them and duly they then become harder on themselves and even abusive upon themselves, never being quite "good enough". They wish to please their parent and get in return love. Often this does not happen. It is healthy for parents to challenge their children but don't over- expect of them. And for children, it is easy to expect unconditional love and support (even financial) from your parents but don't expect this to happen, to such a high degree as may be an impossibility, if so, you just set yourself up for hurt, anger and disappointment.

So to endure family relationships, all parties must thusly lower their expectations of one another to a realistic level and almost one on a friend level. We don't say expect a friend to automatically give us 100 dollars when we need it so why expect this of my mom will be your new thinking. And for parents, stop placing unrealistic goals and "your dreams" upon your child, let them be who they are, an individual, get out of old thinking patterns about who they are (your image in your mind of them) and accept them as they have grown and changed and may have something to actually **teach you**. *Take care of each other.*

We all love our pets in the family, this is easy you know why? because we expect very little from them, they fetch, we are happy and say "good boy", they take a poop and we exclaim "good girl"....easy....they fulfil our lowest expectations and we feel they give so much as it is so easy for pets to love unconditionally as they have no ego, they just exist and are, their purpose is to serve their master, make them happy and they do this easily. As well animals /pets are often predictable whereas humans are unpredictable, this comes into play.

Maybe if we started treating each other in families with the same low expections and just let them be, and be happy with even the littlest accomplishments it would be far more healthy to have these positive and supportive relationships within family makeups/units. Get used to shifted "roles". Remember too high expectations placed on anyone or anything, often can lead to disappointment and all the emotions that go with it. There can be a swirling of emotions too within family from one day being happy, to the next being angry and sad. As hard and challenging as family relationships can be, when successful they can be the most rewarding, so just sit back and be supportive of who each other is and the role they NOW play and hope for a better and healthier future for all. *Love does not hurt, giving it or getting it.*

XV References and Sources

Sources:
-Mainly my own experience having had Fibromyalgia for years
-friends/ Nutritionists/ my original insights thru life & experience
-Dr. Oz show/Iyanla Vazant/ Joel Osteen
-the internet (very little) / TV :

References:

Book: Wheat Belly by Cardiologist William Davis 2012 (USA)

http://www.calmnatural.co.uk/magnesium-deficiency

http://www.ctds.info/magnesium.html (Sandy Simmons)

http://ods.od.nih.gov/factsheet/magnesium-healthprofessional/

http://www.healingwithnutrition.com/fdisease/fibromyalgia/magnesiumstudy.html ("Missing nutrients linked to fibromyalgia and Chronic pain"- by Cathy Leet)

http://www.health-science-spirit.com/magnesiumchloride.html ("Magnesium chloride for health and rejuvenation" by Walter Last)

http://www.aviva.ca/article.asp?articleid=10 ("nutritional protocols and supplements for anxiety" by Nathan Zassman)

http://www.mschachter.com/importance_of_magnesium_to_human.html ("The importance of mg to human nutrition" by Michael Schachter MD FACAM)

http:/www.enerex.ca/en/articles/calcium-to-magnesium-ratio

Randy Peterson- "Changing Ways Clinic", Vancouver BC, **Cda**

"We can never truly let go of how we truly see either our parent or the child, relationships Are fluid however. A true relationship is forever dynamic and changing- growing. We have to have accepting and Open hearts. Believe in one another."

(jemma)

"I'd rather believe in someone and they disappoint me, than not believe and am disappointed in myself"

(jemma)

A book is never finished, alas we can always write another! ..... stay tuned......(this one is 82,000 words and 472,400 characters long)

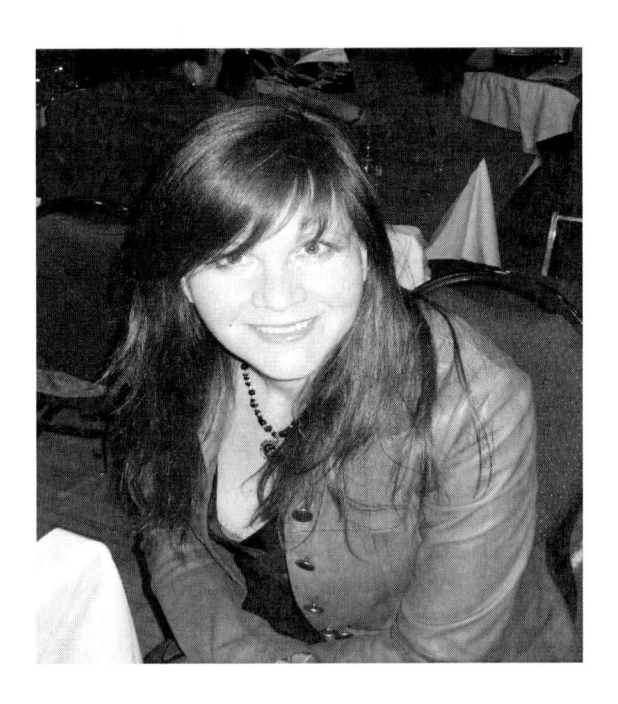

About the Author :

Jemma Jacksen attended the **University of British Columbia** (Canada) in her early 20's where she received a BSc in Agriculture (pre-med). It is here where she obtained her Pre-med sciences and learned all about plant science, animal science and soil science as well as biochemistry, anatomy, genetics, biology and physiology. Later in her mid 20's she fell ill and had many questions why, it took four more years to discover she had a life threatening heart defect she was born with, an ASD (atrial septal defect). It was repaired at age 29, just in the nick of time. From then she abandoned her dreams of one day becoming a doctor and took the path of art for a decade. It was upon an appointment with a wonderful cardiology technologist, while getting an echo of her heart done that she decided to pursue science once again and become a Cardiac Tech. Today she practices both her art and Cardiology Technology (working at a private practice in Canada). She has her BSc (Agr) from UBC and obtained her Diploma in Cardiology Technology, taking courses at both BCIT and a private college in BC, Canada. Throughout her life she experienced alot of illness such as being diagnosed with CFS, Fibromyalgia, ASD (Atrial Septal Defect of the heart), Hypothyroidism, depression and Anaemia to name a few. She was determined through her investigating and learning from others that she was going to resolve her pending health problems and feel better. She has always taken an interest in natural remedies vs. drugs and believed there was an answer. It was through trial and error that she discovered what worked and by investigating it and recording details she has come to write this book, if only to help one other person recover. Jemma experiences great pleasure and reward from helping others in their ailments as well as heart problems. She finds both art and Cardiology very rewarding work indeed and has demonstrated tremendous ability in both. (The front cover of this book is one example of her abstract art work). She looks forward to people, doctors and patients alike and family members of those afflicted with fibromyalgia to gain much from reading her story and of her "cure". Doctors forever never knew what it was, this fibromyalgia, and had a difficult time believing in it besides treating it in those who suffered. It is within these pages that Jemma hopes many will find a wealth of knowledge and exploration into this deeply unknown and unstudied disease called 'Fibromyalgia'. Jemma to this day feels cured and works and lives as tho it never affected her. She hopes you will find the same and go onto live a full and happy life again and help spread the "Cure". With all the questions, mystery and very expensive proclaimed remedies (?) out there, this book is sure to be worth it's weight in gold to anyone who takes an interest.

It is with great thanks that you give it a read, I wish you good health and much success on your path and journey.

(Jemma has an innate passion to help others, especially those suffering, and basically we all can suffer.)

2/3 rds of this book EXPLORES Fibromyalgia (and stress) and the other 1/3 rd discusses Mind, Body, Spirit issues surrounding depression and long term illness.

Contact info:

Fibro Website: **fibrosuccess.com**
(For e- book or to leave stories and inspiration)

to connect with author:
Website:
www.jemmajacksen.com
Email:
info@jemmajacksen.com

or   info@fibrosuccess.com

All Art (& front cover) by Jemma Jacksen :

www.jemmajacksen.com

" A TRUE FRIEND IS ONE WHO CARES ABOUT US EVEN WHEN WE DON'T"   (JEMMA)

"To be wise is to know when you've said enough"

NOTES: